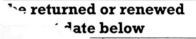

5 minute first aid
for older people

Hodder Arnold

A MEMBER OF THE HODDER HEADLINE GROUP

616.0252

T30310

Orders: Please contact Bookpoint Ltd, 130 Milton Park, Abingdon, Oxon OX14 4SB. Telephone: (44) 01235 827720, Fax: (44) 01235 400454. Lines are open from 9.00 to 18.00, Monday to Saturday, with a 24-hour message answering service. You can also order through our website www.hoddereducation.com

British Library Cataloguing in Publication Data
A catalogue record for this title is available from the British Library.

ISBN-10: 0 340 90463 1
ISBN-13: 9 780340 904633

First published   2005
Impression number   10 9 8 7 6 5 4 3 2 1
Year   2008 2007 2006 2005

Typeset by Transet Limited, Coventry, England.
Printed in Great Britain for Hodder Arnold, a division of Hodder Headline, 338 Euston Road, London NW1 3BH, by Cox & Wyman Ltd, Reading, Berkshire.

Hodder Headline's policy is to use papers that are natural, renewable and recyclable products and made from wood grown in sustainable forests. The logging and manufacturing processes are expected to conform to the environmental regulations of the country of origin.

contents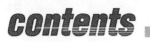

acknowledgements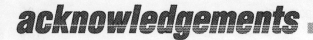

The authors would like to pay special thanks to Charlotte Hall, Catherine Jones, Teresa Mulligan, Genevieve Okech and Naomi Safir.

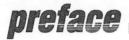

preface

The British Red Cross, as part of the International Red Cross and Red Crescent Movement, is the world's largest first-aid training organization. With over 180 Red Cross societies worldwide we endeavour to make first-aid knowledge and skills accessible to individuals, families, schools and the wider community.

You never know when someone may need your help but it is highly likely that when called on to provide emergency first aid it will be to someone close to you such as a friend or a member of your own family. Therefore, we have produced the *Five-minute First Aid* series in order to give you the relevant skills and confidence needed to be able to save a life and help an injured person, whatever your situation.

We appreciate that it is difficult to find time in hectic lifestyles to learn first-aid skills. Consequently, this series is designed so that you can learn and absorb each specific, essential skill that is relevant to you in just five minutes, and you can pick up and put down the book as you wish. The features throughout the book will help you to reinforce what you have learnt and will build your confidence in applying first aid.

This book is divided into five-minute sections, so that you can discover each invaluable skill in just a short amount of time.

---

one-minute wonder

One-minute wonders ask and answer the questions that you might be thinking as you read.

---

 key skills

The key-skill features emphasize and reiterate the main skills of the section – helping you to commit them to memory and recall them when called upon to do so.

summary

Summary sections summarize the key points of the chapter in order to further consolidate your knowledge and understanding.

self-testers

The self-testers ensure that you have learnt the most important facts of the chapter. They will give you an indication of how much you are absorbing as you go along and help to build your confidence. (Note: some of the multiple choice questions may have more than one possible answer!)

We hope that this book will give you the opportunity to learn the most important skills you will ever need in a friendly, straightforward way, and that it prepares you for any first-aid situation that you may encounter.

introduction

This book offers you an insight into the most common injuries and conditions that may affect the older members of our society. We all recognize that as we get older the risk of illness and injury increases, and in this book we not only highlight the most common situations you may encounter that require first aid but also offer specific advice on what you should do. Most people think many of the situations described in this book will not happen to them, but the reality is that most of us will become injured or unwell at some point in our lives. Even if we are fortunate and this does not happen to us until later in life, we are likely to encounter a situation where your first-aid skills could, in the most serious cases, make the difference between life and death. In the more routine situations it can reduce a person's discomfort and speed up their recovery.

In recent years we have gained a greater understanding of the importance of the initial care a person receives in the minutes after an accident, and in this book we focus on the key things that will make a difference. Much of the content may appear to be common sense, such as if a person is not breathing you must breathe for him, or if his heart is not working you must simulate the work of the heart. Nevertheless, how you do these things and the order in which you do them are very important. We also make reference throughout the book to what we call 'psychological first aid' – a complex term that simply means talking to and reassuring the person while you are treating them.

This book describes how to assess a person's injuries, tells you what you should do in a logical and simple way, and answers the most common questions that are asked in relation to each subject.

While we are confident that this book contains all the information and advice to help you deal with the most common emergencies involving older people, we know that these are only of value if you are prepared to help and to use the information and advice if called upon to do so. Don't be a bystander, don't assume someone else will do something – get involved.

We have tried to make first aid simple, practical and easy to understand. Try not to be one of the many people who mean to learn first aid but don't get around to it until it's too late. We know that most people who require first aid are treated by someone who knows them. That person could be you.

For convenience and clarity, we use the pronoun 'he' when referring to the first aider or injured person.

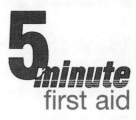

1

how to deal with an emergency

Accidents, injuries and sudden illness are unavoidable, however as you get older, the risk of an accident, injury and illness increases. Many of us who are involved in the care of an older person or are old ourselves feel unprepared to help in an emergency situation. There is a variety of reasons for this. The most common reason is the idea that 'it won't happen to me'; other reasons include not wanting to get involved, assuming someone else will deal with it, or simply a lack of skills and knowledge about what to do. We all know there is no way of predicting when and where we may be called upon to help and therefore the sense of being unprepared is understandable. However, as you will find out by reading this book, there are some simple things you can do while waiting for the ambulance or the doctor to arrive. In a few situations your actions may save the person's life, and on other occasions you can prevent his condition from deteriorating, or you may speed up the person's recovery.

If you are a relative, friend or carer of an older person it is very likely that one day you will have to deal with an emergency situation, and so it is important for you to be aware of what to do.

⑤ ● ⑤

an emergency situation

When you find yourself dealing with an unexpected emergency situation you must make sure you are not putting yourself in danger. If there is obvious danger, call the emergency services and wait for them to arrive before approaching the incident. There is a range of things that may pose a risk to you when dealing with an emergency situation. The more common ones are listed on page 23.

The ultimate decision about whether to help rests with you, but remember you will not be in a position to help anyone if you end up injured yourself. It is also important to keep bystanders away from the danger, so warn them if you can. We in the British Red Cross have been delivering first aid for more than 100 years, and we know that first-aid incidents in public places attract a large number of onlookers, many of whom are prepared to get involved and help you. Some of these situations are poorly handled because no one has stepped forward and demonstrated any leadership qualities, assessed the danger, delegated responsibility or delivered some immediate care.

calling for help

First-aid incidents can happen anywhere at any time, in any weather and often when least expected. In the case of an older person this can be in the home, in the garden or on the road, to name a few examples. Each of these settings brings a unique set of challenges to you if you are the first person on the scene. No one expects you to cope on your own – you will need help from onlookers, neighbours, and eventually from the emergency services if the situation is serious.

Everyone, when faced with an emergency, feels some anxiety, irrespective of how much training he has had. As soon as you think there is the prospect of dealing with an emergency, however large or small, it is a good idea to shout loudly to see if anyone can come to help. You will feel less anxious if you have help. You may also have to do several tasks at once, such as ensuring that the area around you and the injured person(s) is safe, and calling for the emergency services – it is better if you have someone to help. This appears obvious, but when you feel anxious it is easy to forget. Instruct a bystander to help you and advise him about what to do, for example, bringing first-aid equipment including a blanket and a first-aid kit. You will read more about how this equipment should be used later in the book. It is also important to maintain a person's privacy (only remove clothing and expose the person if necessary). Help to administer first aid.

Anyone who is with you can be helpful if given clear instructions about what to do. If people are kept busy, it may reduce the panic and confusion that always surrounds a significant emergency.

You may be the most experienced or confident first aider present, and of course often you will be the only person present. Take control, tell others you have some first-aid knowledge and try to keep a clear picture of what is happening so that you can pass on accurate information to the emergency services. If you ask a bystander to call the emergency services, make sure it is done.

calling the emergency services

To call the emergency services in the UK you must dial 999; in the European Union dial 112. Both numbers will put you through to the operator.

When you dial 999 you will be asked which service you require. If it is a significant emergency with several injured people or if safety is a problem, you will need fire, police and ambulance.

The operator will ask you for some information about the emergency, so it is important to know some answers before you phone, such as your location and your phone number. You will also be asked to give an indication of the type and seriousness of the emergency, the number of people injured, and whether or not there are any dangers such as chemicals or toxic fumes.

(5) • (5)

managing an incident

It is important to adopt a systematic approach to any emergency in order to give the injured people the best chance of survival. Make sure you are clear in your mind about how to use bystanders, how to access the emergency services and how to assess the people for injuries.

 key skills

Dial 999 or 112. Remember the location of the accident, how many people are involved and some basic information about the extent of their injuries or illnesses.

assessing the scene for injured people

Make sure you know how many people are involved. Check the quiet ones first because they may be unconscious and will need your attention first. You can be sure that if a person is shouting or crying out in pain he is not unconscious and not in immediate danger. Ask helpers to remove from the scene any people with minor injuries to improve access to those with serious injuries.

Perform an initial assessment known as the 'primary survey' on any unconscious people and prioritize the treatment of any unconscious people (see below). Treat conscious people with serious injuries first, then treat conscious people with less serious injuries.

In the following pages we describe the levels of assessment you can carry out when attempting to find out what injuries or illness a person may have. In many situations the injuries or conditions will be obvious and will not require this level of assessment. However, you may come across circumstances, for example, a car accident, where there is more than one injured person and you are going to have to treat the injured in order of priority. On other occasions the person's injury or illness may not be obvious.

⑤ • ⑤

the primary survey

The aim of the primary survey is to establish if the person is conscious and breathing. Based on your findings you can decide if life-saving first aid is needed.

You should already know if there is any danger to you or the injured person from your assessment of the incident scene. Only after making sure it is safe to do so, find out whether the person is conscious or unconscious. To do this, shout loudly. Call the person's name if you know it; if you do not get an obvious reaction, shake the shoulders gently. If you still do not get a response, assume the person is unconscious. If the person is unconscious and you have not already shouted for help do that now.

If the person is unconscious, you should then open the airway. To do this you first place one hand on the forehead and gently tilt the head back. This will make the mouth fall open so that you can look for any obvious obstruction to the airway in or around the mouth and, if present, remove it. Then place two fingers under the point of the chin and lift. This will open the airway.

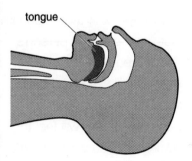

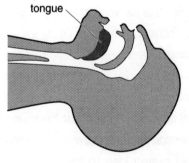

(a) Blocked airway – head not tilted   (b) Unblocked airway – head tilted

Fig 1 Importance of an open airway

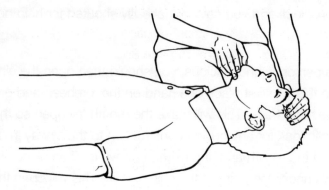

Fig 2 To open the airway
Place one hand on the forehead and your fingertips under the chin and gently tilt the head back.

With the airway open, you can now check to see if the person is breathing. You do this by lowering your head over the person's mouth and nose. Look, listen and feel for breathing for around ten seconds. If the person is breathing you will see the chest moving up and down. Always look towards the person's toes otherwise you will not be able to see the chest. You will feel the person's breath on your cheek, but remember you will have to get quite close to the mouth and nose to do this. You will hear the sound of the person's breathing. If you are in a noisy place like a busy road, it can be very difficult to hear a person breathing. You may have to rely on observing the chest for movement and feeling for breath on your cheek.

If the person is breathing, look for any other life-threatening injuries such as severe bleeding. If there is severe bleeding you will be able to see it without searching around and moving the person. If present, you should treat it. If there are no other life-threatening injuries, the safest position for the person is the recovery position (Chapter 2, page 36).

 key skills

To open the airway of an unconscious person you should place one hand on the forehead and gently tilt the head back. Then place two fingers under the point of the chin and lift.

assessing the injuries

Before moving the person into the recovery position, you should consider whether or not there is likely to be an injury to the neck. To do this, look at the mechanism of the injury – this is a term we use to describe the detail of the accident. Unless you witness an accident you will have to make assumptions about how the person ended up as he did, and this may then give you an indication of possible injuries. For example, if the person has been thrown from a moving vehicle and hit his head, it is likely there will be a neck injury. In this instance it may be better to leave the person in the position in which you found him and maintain an open airway using the jaw-thrust technique (see Figure 3).

In this circumstance, whether or not to move the person into the recovery position can be a difficult decision to make. If the airway can be maintained using the jaw thrust that is good, but if you can't maintain the airway or the person shows any sign of vomiting then you must turn him into the recovery position. If you have a helper you can ask him to steady the head (see Figure 4) while you turn the person into the recovery position (Chapter 2, page 36).

---

one-minute *wonder*

Q When I am deciding whether or not to turn the person into the recovery position, which takes priority, a possible neck injury or an open and clear airway?

A An open and clear airway takes priority over other injuries because if the airway is not open the person cannot breathe and if a person cannot breathe he will die.

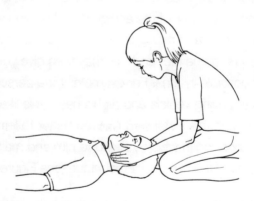

Fig 3 The jaw-thrust technique

Gently lift the jaw to open the airway.

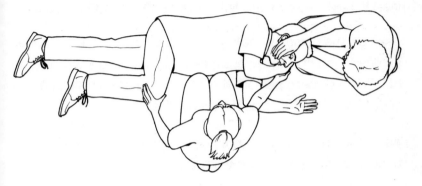

Fig 4 Turning the person into the recovery position

the secondary survey

Having completed the primary survey and decided that no life-saving action is required, you can do a 'secondary survey'. The aim of the secondary survey is to find out more about the person's condition so that the correct first aid can be administered.

You should find out more about the incident by talking to the person and any bystanders. Ask what happened, when it happened, where it happened and possibly why it happened. Consider the mechanism of the injury by looking at how the incident occurred. For example, in a car crash if the impact is from the side, injuries are likely to be on that side of the body.

Ask how the person is feeling. He may be able to tell you about an illness and how the illness makes him feel. A good example of this is a diabetic person who can tell you when his blood sugar is low and how this makes him feel.

Assess the person's injuries by examining him and carrying out a 'head-to-toe survey' (see below).

⑤ ● ⑤

the head-to-toe survey

As the title implies, the head-to-toe survey involves checking the injured person in some detail, from the top of the head to the feet.

So that you don't miss any vital clues about a person's injuries, it is best to be systematic when doing this: start from the head and work down the body to the toes. Place your hands on the person's body and feel for any abnormal swelling or tenderness. Very often it is not possible to make a definite diagnosis without tests that are only available in hospital, but it is possible to suspect an injury or illness and give the correct first-aid treatment.

You can gain more information about the problem by looking for external clues. For example, objects that could have caused injury, a warning bracelet giving medical history, a card indicating diabetes, allergy or epilepsy, an inhaler that may indicate breathing problems, and medicines such as Glyceryl TriNitrate (GTN) which indicate a history of angina – a common problem in older people.

You should then look for general signs and symptoms. The term 'signs and symptoms' is used widely in first aid. Signs refer to what you can see – blood loss and skin colour are two of the more common signs. Symptoms are what the injured or ill person feels and examples include pain and tenderness. It is also important to ask the injured person about their symptoms and of course listen to what they tell you.

Ask the person if he has pain anywhere. If the answer is yes, look at that area for injury. Check the quality of the breathing, it may be fast, slow or laboured, The term 'laboured' means the injured person is having difficulty breathing in and out. These signs and symptoms may indicate that the person has a chest injury. Check the quality of the pulse (see page 14). It may be fast; the normal pulse rate in an adult is between 60 and 80 beats per minute but it may be up to 100 beats per minutes in an older person. It is not unusual for an injured person to have a high pulse rate due to the traumatic events he has been involved in, but it can also indicate a possible heart condition or blood loss. It is important to continue to monitor the pulse while waiting for the ambulance to see if it is getting faster or slower. The pulse may also be regular or irregular. 'Irregular' is used to describe a pulse that has different intervals between each beat. If this is the case, the person may have a heart problem. Look at the skin as there may be blueness around the lips. Blueness may indicate that the person has breathing difficulties. Feel the skin – it may be cold and clammy, and the person may be suffering from shock.

⑤ • ⑤

how to take the pulse

A pulse is the impact felt from the wave of blood as it flows through a person's arteries. There are many points in the body where you can find a pulse, but the most common places to take a pulse are at the wrist and in the neck.

To take the pulse at the wrist, place two fingers at the base of the thumb just below the wrist creases. To take the pulse in the neck, place two fingers on the side of the neck between the windpipe and the large muscle in the neck.

Assess whether the pulse is fast or slow, weak or strong, regular or irregular, remembering that the normal rate in an average adult is between 60 and 80 beats per minute but that it may be up to 100 per minute in an older person. Ask the person if he knows his usual pulse rate.

(a) By the wrist

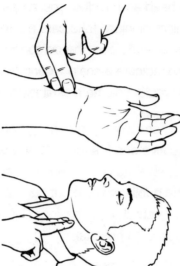

(b) By the neck

Fig 5 Taking the pulse

 key skills

Always look for external clues as to what may have caused the injury and any other information on the person that may help the treatment.

one-minute wonder

Q If I am assessing a person and I find that he has cold, clammy skin and a fast, weak pulse, what should I suspect?

A Shock.

Look around the head and neck. If you suspect a neck injury from the mechanism of injury, take care not to move the head. Move your hands carefully over the person's head. Feel for blood – this would indicate a scalp wound. Feel for a depression in the skull – this would indicate a skull fracture.

Look for any blood or yellow fluid coming from the nose or the ears – this is indicative of a fracture of the skull. Look for bleeding, bruising, swelling or a foreign object in the eyes; look at the pupils. If the pupils are different sizes after a head injury, this may indicate cerebral compression. This is a condition that needs early admission to hospital.

Look for swelling, bleeding or bruising around the mouth and smell the person's breath. You may notice alcohol or a smell like pear drop sweets; if it does smell like pear drops this may indicate that the person has a diabetic problem (see Chapter 6, page 96). Look at the neck and wrists for a medical warning necklace or wrist bracelet; these are worn by a large number of older people who have relevant medical conditions.

Feel along both collarbones for fractures or dislocations.

Look at the chest, the back and the abdomen. Ask the person if he has any back pain. If back pain is accompanied by problems in moving the legs, numbness or tingling, do not allow the person to move in case there is a serious back injury. Any unnecessary movement may result in permanent damage.

Look at the chest for wounds and ask the person to take a deep breath, and watch the movement. If there is unequal movement – by this we mean if one side of the chest is rising and the other side is not moving to the same extent – there may be a chest injury.

Listen for wheezing. This may indicate breathing problems. Check for wounds, swelling, bruising or bleeding around the chest or abdomen. Feel the abdomen for any tenderness or muscle rigidity that may indicate an internal injury.

Look for incontinence; this may indicate that the person has had a seizure. Examine the pelvis for deformity, as this may indicate a fracture.

Look at the limbs and check for any wounds, swelling, bruising, bleeding or deformity. Look for needle marks, a medical warning necklace or bracelet and look at the nails for blueness as this may show that the person is cold.

⑤ ● ⑤

monitoring vital signs

You have carried out the primary survey to assess whether or not life-saving measures are required, and you have carried out the secondary and head-to-toe surveys to try to find out the problem.

Having given the correct first-aid treatment, you should now take some baseline measurements of breathing, pulse and level of response while waiting for the emergency services to arrive. If possible you should take these measurements regularly and record them because they can be used to monitor whether a person's condition is getting better or worse. We have already covered how to take a pulse as part of the head-to-toe survey.

how to check the breathing

Listen to the person's breaths and watch the chest rise and fall. Try to do this without the person realizing because we are all able to voluntarily control our breathing. Listen for wheezing or breathing difficulties.

Assess whether the breathing is fast or slow, deep or shallow, easy, difficult or painful. Remember that the normal rate in an average adult is between 12 and 16 breaths per minute.

how to check the level of response

To monitor the level of response of an unconscious person, we use a process called AVPU – each letter refers to the level of a person's consciousness.

Alert   Is the person alert and behaving normally?

Verbal   Is the person responding to your voice and able to answer simple questions and obey simple commands?

Pain   Does the person open his eyes or move if pinched?

Unconscious   Is the person not responding to any stimuli?

cross-infection, shock and post-emergency anxiety

Other things to watch out for when dealing with an emergency include:

- the risk and dangers of cross-infection
- the presence of shock
- the anxiety you will feel when the emergency is over.

the risks of cross-infection

In any situation when you are dealing with other people there is a potential risk of transferring infective organisms such as viruses and bacteria from one person to another. This is especially possible when dealing with body fluids, particularly blood and other body fluids contaminated with blood. It is wise, therefore, to take some simple precautions. Wash your hands if possible before and after each contact and wear disposable gloves if you can, but if gloves are not available do not hold back from life saving. Use the person's own hands to put pressure on a bleeding wound. If you do not have gloves you can cover your hands with clean plastic bags and cover any wounds you have on your hands with waterproof dressings.

Try to avoid blood splashes in your eyes or mouth. If you are splashed in the eye, nose, mouth or in a skin wound, wash thoroughly and seek advice from your doctor. Use a plastic bag to dispose of any soiled rubbish and tie it securely around the top.

the presence of shock

'Shock' is a term used to describe a range of situations from feelings of anxiety to a serious clinical state in which the body has lost a lot of blood or body fluids, and it is important to be aware of the differences. In all emergency situations there will be a feeling of shock and anxiety about what has happened.

Clinical shock is common after injury and is a life-threatening state in which the circulating fluid in the body is reduced and organs such as the heart and brain do not get enough blood and therefore there is not enough oxygen and nutrients for them to function properly. It is most commonly the result of blood loss but it can be caused by fluid loss, as in burns.

If you suspect shock you should look for pale, cold, clammy skin, restlessness, yawning, sighing, nausea and thirst, rapid and then weak pulse, fast and shallow breathing, and gradual loss of consciousness.

To help a person in shock you should treat the underlying problem if possible. Help the person to lie down and reassure constantly, as he will be very anxious. Raise the legs above the level of the heart so that the blood in the legs flows down towards the heart and the brain where it is most needed. Keep the person warm by covering with a light blanket, but remember overheating will make the shock worse.

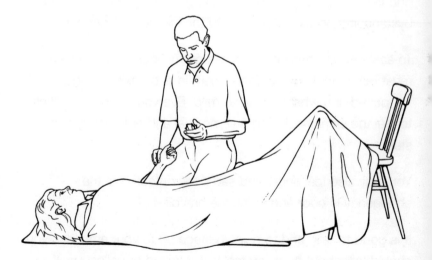

Fig 6 Treating a person in shock

Monitor and record the pulse, breathing and level of response regularly until help arrives. Do not give the person anything to eat or drink as further treatment requiring an anaesthetic may be necessary in hospital.

the anxiety you will feel when the emergency is over

An emergency is a distressing experience for everyone involved. When you are dealing with the problems you will be active and focused on what you are doing. However, when it is over and the emergency services have taken the people to hospital and have cleared up, this is the time when you are likely to start asking yourself questions like, did I do the correct things?; Did I phone for help early enough?; Did I get enough help from the bystanders?; What will happen to the injured or ill people?

To ask yourself these questions is normal behaviour and you must realize that you will feel uncertain and anxious about what happened and what you did to help. Everyone involved is likely to feel the same, including any medical and emergency services staff.

You may also feel angry and sad if the outcome of the emergency is poor and someone has died.

It is good to talk, and to help you face up to your emotions you should talk about how you feel with a friend or colleague. It would be very beneficial to talk to someone else who was involved in the emergency so that you can share feelings. Confidentiality is important so you should not refer to people involved in the emergency by name or other personal identification when talking, but there is no reason why you can't talk about your feelings.

If you release your feelings soon after the emergency you will probably be able to cope more easily than if you keep your feelings to yourself. Nonetheless, you may still experience feelings of anxiety for some time after the event. These may include flashbacks of what happened, nightmares or disturbed sleep, sweating and tremors, nausea, (especially when thinking about what happened), tension and irritability, and feelings of isolation and lack of self-confidence. If you continue to suffer from any of these problems you should ask for help from your doctor.

⑤ ● ⑤

is it too risky to help?

Every emergency situation presents you with a unique set of challenges and there may be occasions when it will be too dangerous for you to become involved. When assessing an emergency situation, it is important to consider the risks that exist at the time and any other potential risks that may occur when managing the incident.

We have detailed some of the common situations you may be required to respond to and highlighted some of the potential risks you may want to consider below.

smoke, fire and flames

It is often the smoke that kills rather than the fire. Also, check for the presence of the toxic fumes or hazardous chemicals particularly in road traffic accidents. Other situations that may be dangerous include bomb blasts and falling masonry. Rescuing people from water presents you, the rescuer, with many potential dangers, especially if you are a non-swimmer. Dangers include deep water, very cold water or flood water.

If there is no serious danger and you think it is safe to approach an incident, try to find out what has happened.

⑤ ● ⑤

specific incidents

car crash

If you come across a car crash and it is safe to approach, park your vehicle safely, switch on your hazard lights and alert the emergency services. At a car crash you will usually need police, fire and ambulance services. Use your warning triangles to alert other road users, by placing them on the side of the road where other drivers can see them. They should be at least 45 m away from the crash in either direction. Send bystanders to warn other drivers. Stabilize any vehicles involved in the crash by switching off the ignition and applying the handbrake. Make sure you look for all the people involved; car accident victims are often found in unusual places, some distance from the scene of the original accident.

🌐 *key skills*

When dealing with any accident, and in particular a road traffic accident, ensure that the scene is safe, assess the number and potential severity of the injuries to the people involved. Dial 999 (or 112 in Europe) for the emergency services and begin treatment, dealing with the most severely injured first.

one-minute *wonder*

Q If I am treating a person in the middle of the road should I move him first?

A It is important that you do not move the person until you have assessed his injuries. Even then, if you suspect a back or neck injury you must not move the person. Instead, ask bystanders to stop the traffic.

fire

If you are aware of a fire or of smoke, sound the fire alarm and warn as many people as possible in the area of the fire. Remember that fire and smoke can spread quickly. There are some general principles to follow:

- if the fire is small and you have a fire blanket or fire extinguisher, you can try to put out the fire, but do not try for longer than 30 seconds
- if the fire has taken hold, do not try to put it out, do not use lifts, and close all doors behind you
- do not open a door without first touching the door handle with the back of your hand. If it is hot this indicates there is a fire behind the door so do not open it but instead find another escape route
- walk quickly but do not run. If you have to cross a smoke-filled area, stay close to the ground where there will be the least smoke
- if trapped by a fire, go into a room with a window and shut the door. Open the window and shout for help. If you are able to reach the ground outside the building from the window, escape by going out feet first and lowering yourself onto the ground. Call the emergency services as soon as possible.

If you have to deal with a person whose clothes are on fire you should stop, drop, wrap and roll:

- **stop** the person from moving around, as this will make the fire worse
- **drop** the person to the ground
- **wrap** the person in a non-flammable material.
- **roll** the person slowly along the ground to extinguish the flames.

To treat the person for burns, see Chapter 9, page 134.

 key skills

If you have to deal with a person whose clothes are on fire, you should get him to stop, drop, wrap and roll.

water

The main dangers relating to rescue from water are that the water may be cold, deep and there may be strong underwater currents. When attempting to rescue someone from water it is very important that you do not put yourself at risk. It is best to rescue from the water's edge, making sure that you do not get pulled into the water. You can throw a rope or a float to the person, or reach out with a stick or branch if he is close to the edge.

If you have to go into the water, wade rather than swim and do not go out of your depth. Make sure the person's head is out of the water and then drag him to the side. Do not lift him unnecessarily. Try to shield the person from cold wind to prevent any further hypothermia.

electricity

The majority of injuries caused by an electric current are due to faulty switches or appliances. We have become increasingly aware of electrocution as a result of people using DIY tools and electric lawnmowers. The possiblity of water or wet grass being present makes this situation more potentially hazardous.

When dealing with an electrical incident you must never touch the person until he is isolated from the electrical current because if you make contact with the current you too will be electrocuted.

You should, if possible, switch off the electricity at the socket. If this is not possible, separate the person from the electrical source. To do this, stand on some dry, insulating material such as a book or folded newspaper, then use something made of wood such as a broom to push the electrical source away from the person or the person away from the source. If this is still not possible, carefully loop some rope around the person's ankles and pull him away from the source.

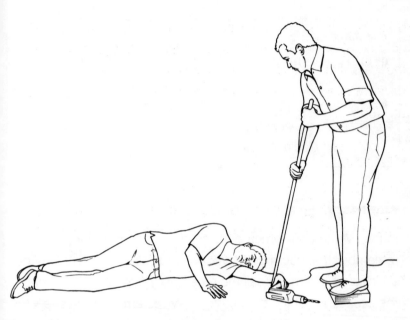

Fig 7 Breaking the person's contact with the source of electricity

---

one-minute wonder

Q Why do you advise that water may present a risk to a first aider responding to a DIY accident?

A Many electrocution incidents involving DIY, result from the person drilling through a live electric cable or through a water pipe with water coming in contact with the electrical components of the drill. As water conducts electricity, you should be extremely cautious when dealing with this type of incident.

***one-minute** wonder*

Q Can I use a metal pole to isolate the person from the electricity?

A Unfortunately metal will conduct electricity and you will receive a shock, so you must use a material that does not conduct electricity, such as wood or paper.

---

summary

In the event of any emergency situation, it is important to remember that you must never put yourself in danger. Carry out an initial assessment, call the emergency services and manage the situation until the emergency services arrive. Always talk to and listen to the injured person, giving lots of reassurance.

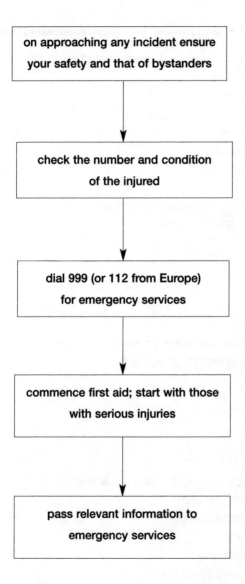

on approaching any incident ensure
your safety and that of bystanders

↓

check the number and condition
of the injured

↓

dial 999 (or 112 from Europe)
for emergency services

↓

commence first aid; start with those
with serious injuries

↓

pass relevant information to
emergency services

Dealing with an emergency

self-testers ▬▬▬▬▬▬▬▬▬▬▬▬▬▬▬▬▬▬▬▬

1 Which of the following dangers will stop you from approaching an emergency?
   a toxic fumes
   b swimming pool of water
   c bomb blast
   d moving vehicles
   e falling masonry

2 When dealing with a person whose clothes are on fire, what do the following letters stand for?
   S _____
   D _____
   W _____
   R _____

3 When you are monitoring a person's level of reponse, what do the following letters stand for?
   A _____
   V _____
   P _____
   U _____

4 Which of the following indicate clinical shock?
   a cold, clammy skin
   b strong, slow pulse
   c thirst
   d slow breathing
   e sighing and yawning

5 **Which of the following are actions taken to treat clinical shock?**
   a taking the person's clothes off
   b raising the head and shoulders
   c treating the underlying cause
   d standing the person up
   e raising the person's legs

6 **Which of the following will reduce the chance of cross-infection?**
   a washing your hands after dealing with another person
   b putting a waterproof dressing on the cut on your hand
   c avoiding splashes of blood getting in your eye
   d wearing disposable gloves
   e disposing of all soiled rubbish in a sealed plastic bag

answers
1 **a**, **c** and **e**
2 **S**top, **D**rop, **W**rap and **R**oll
3 **A**lert, **V**erbal, **P**ain, **U**nconscious
4 **a**, **c** and **e**
5 **c** and **e**
6 **a**, **b**, **c**, **d** and **e**

2

how to resuscitate

Finding a person collapsed and in need of resuscitation is a frightening experience, and so it is important to try to remain calm and think clearly. You should know when to call an ambulance and be ready to give the ambulance service personnel an indication of the urgency of the situation. This is important as most ambulance services prioritize calls based on the information the caller gives them. If the person is not breathing you will need to breathe for him. If there are no signs of heart activity you will need to do chest compressions.

In this chapter you will learn how to check for a response, how to check for breathing and how to do chest compressions. You will also be advised as to the best time to call an ambulance.

In Chapter 1 you were given information about dangers that you might encounter such as electricity and fire, and therefore in this chapter we will assume that any obvious danger has been dealt with.

⑤ • ⑤

checking for a response

To check for a response, talk to the person, call his name if you know it and gently shake his shoulders. Remember that if you do this too vigorously you may cause an injury, especially to the neck. If there is no response, shout for help and open the airway as described in Chapter 1 (page 7).

 key skills

In order for a person to breathe, he needs to have an open airway. This can be achieved by lifting the chin and tilting the head back.

---

one-minute *wonder*

Q Should dentures always be removed?

A Not necessarily. If dentures are dislodged, then remove them but if they are fitting well and are in place, leave them.

is the person breathing?

When the airway is open, ask yourself 'Is the person breathing?' Check for breathing as described in Chapter 1 (page 18).

key skills

Look, listen and feel for breathing.

---

one-minute wonder

Q People often talk of swallowing the tongue. What does this
  mean?
A The tongue is not actually swallowed, but when you lose
  consciousness you also lose muscle tone and if you are
  lying on your back the tongue can flop into the back of the
  throat and block the airway. When you tip the head back the
  tongue regains its normal position in the floor of the mouth.

If the person is breathing look for any other life-threatening
problems such as severe bleeding. Deal with these problems
then place the person in the recovery position.

⑤ ● ⑤

the recovery position

The recovery position is the safest position for an unconscious
person to be in. It ensures that the tongue does not block the
airway, any vomit drains from the mouth and if there is any
blood in the throat it drains out and does not stop the person
from breathing.

To place a person in the recovery position, kneel beside him and remove spectacles and any bulky objects from the pocket on the side you are going to roll him onto. Place the arm that is nearest to you in the 'How' position at the shoulder. Bring the other arm across the body and hold the back of this hand against the person's cheek. With your other hand, grasp the far leg just above the knee and pull it up until the foot is flat on the floor. Pull on the far leg and roll the person towards you. Adjust the upper leg so that it is at right angles at the hip and the knee. Tilt the person's head back to make sure the airway stays open.

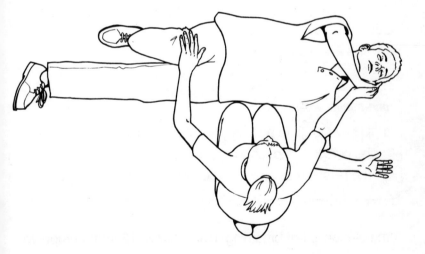

Fig 8 Rolling the injured person into the recovery position

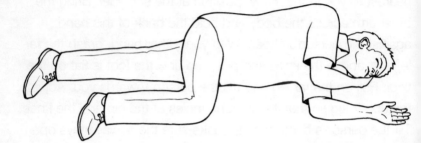

Fig 9 The finished recovery position

---

one-minute wonder

Q If I have to go to a telephone to get help, is it safe to leave
   the person in the recovery position?

A The person is as safe as is possible in the recovery position.

If the person is not breathing, dial 999 (or 112 from Europe) for
emergency help and then give two rescue breaths.

ⓢ • ⓢ

rescue breaths – the 'kiss of life'

Keeping the airway open, pinch the nose and place your mouth around the person's mouth. Blow steadily until the chest rises, then take your mouth away and watch the chest fall. If the chest rises as you blow and falls as you take your mouth away, you have given an effective breath.

Having called for emergency help and given two effective rescue breaths, ask yourself 'Does this person have any signs of blood circulation?' The signs are breathing, coughing, eye opening or movement of the body or limbs. Take a quick look for no longer than ten seconds. In the older person it is unlikely there will be signs so you should try to provide some artificial blood circulation by doing chest compressions; you may be more familiar with the terms 'chest thumps' or 'heart massage'. Nowadays we tend to use the term 'chest compressions' to describe the technique that simulates the work of the heart to get some blood around the body (see page 41).

---

one-minute wonder

Q I thought that checking to see whether the person had a pulse was the best way to see if the person has a blood circulation.

A Checking the pulse is one way to see if the person has a circulation, but we now know that finding a pulse in an older person who has collapsed is very difficult. Our advice is don't delay in trying to locate a pulse, look for obvious signs of circulation as described above.

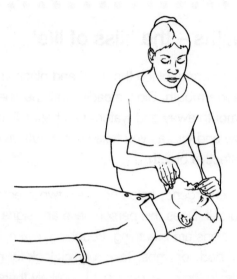

(a) Tilt the head back and pinch the nose.

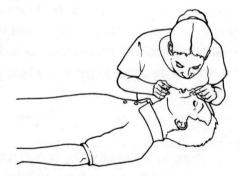

(b) Place your mouth over the person's mouth and blow.

Fig 10 How to give rescue breaths

key skills

To deliver rescue breaths, open the airway, pinch the nose and blow into the collapsed person's mouth until you see the chest rise.

---

one-minute wonder

Q If the older person is breathing and I do rescue breathing will I smother him?

A No, the chances of smothering someone in this way are very slim and the benefits of saving a life using this procedure far outweighs this concern.

⑤ • ⑤

chest compressions

Kneel beside the person and find the lower part of the breastbone. Do this by using your middle finger of one hand to find the point where the lowermost rib meets the breastbone. Place your index finger on the breastbone beside your middle finger, run the heel of your other hand down the breastbone and place it next to the fingers. This is the point you apply pressure.

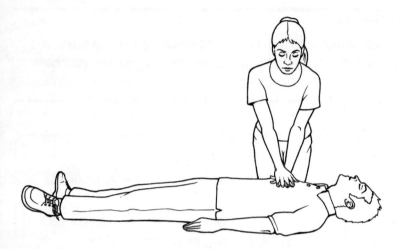

Fig 11 How to do chest compressions
Keep your arms straight and use the heel of your hand to press down.

Place the heel of one hand on the breastbone, then place the heel of your other hand on top and interlock your fingers. Lean over the person and, keeping your arms straight, press down by about 4–5 cm (1.5–2 inches) at a rate of 100 per minute. Release the pressure without taking your hands off the chest.

Combine chest compressions with rescue breaths at a ratio of two breaths to 15 chest compressions. This is CPR – cardio pulmonary resuscitation. Continue CPR until help arrives and takes over, or until you are so exhausted that you cannot carry on, or until the person takes a breath or makes a movement.

🕐 *key skills*

The ratio of rescue breaths to chest compressions for an adult is two breaths followed by 15 compressions. The aim of chest compressions is not to restart the heart. To do this you need a piece of equipment called a defibrillator which sends an electrical charge across the heart. The aim of chest compressions is to maintain some blood circulation while waiting for the emergency services to arrive.

one-minute wonder

Q A friend told me that if you do chest compressions on an older person you may break his ribs?

A There is a risk of fracturing ribs as a result of pressing on the chest, but please do not let this be a deterrent to attempting to save someone's life.

one-minute wonder

Q Is it possible for a person to stop breathing but to still have a heartbeat?

A It is possible, but in the older person it is more likely that the problem causing the collapse is related to the heart and therefore it is likely that the heart has stopped.

summary

If you come across an incident where somebody requires resuscitation, try to think quickly and logically. Call an ambulance, commence CPR and try to stay as calm as possible.

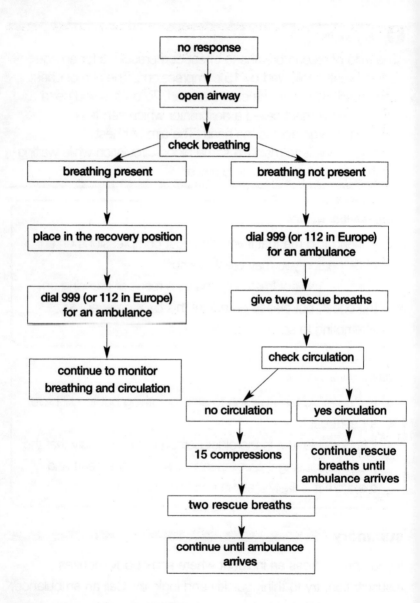

How to assess an unconcious person

self-testers

1 The recovery position is a safe position because:
   a if the person is sick the vomit will drain away
   b the airway stays open
   c the person can easily roll onto his back
   d the tongue doesn't drop back into the throat
   e the chest moves freely

2 When looking for signs of circulation what do you check for?
   a moving
   b eye opening
   c skin colour
   d breathing
   e coughing

3 What is the ratio of rescue breaths to chest compressions?
   a 2:15
   b 1:5
   c 2:10
   d 3:12
   e 4:20

4 What is the rate for chest compressions?
   a 80 per minute
   b as fast as you can
   c 100 per minute
   d it changes for people of different sizes
   e it changes for people of different ages

5 **When checking for a response what should you do?**
  a hit the person between the shoulder blades
  b speak loudly and clearly
  c use the person's name if you know it
  d shake the shoulders gently
  e stamp your feet around the person's head

answers
1 **a**, **b**, **d** and **e**
2 **a**, **b**, **d** and **e**
3 **a**
4 **c**
5 **b**, **c** and **d**

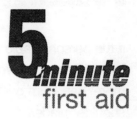

3

choking

Choking happens when a person has something stuck in the throat. The object is frequently a piece of food such as a fish bone or a hard piece of meat. If an older person is particularly frail this will make the efforts to cough up the object more difficult and so choking can rapidly turn into an emergency situation.

how to deal with choking

It is important to recognize that when a person is choking you must take prompt action, as he may not be able to alert you by calling out. The signs that will make you suspect someone is choking include coughing, difficulty breathing and clutching the throat. You may also suspect choking from the fact that the person is eating or has just been eating. A choking episode can be very frightening as well as embarrassing.

If the person is able to cough encourage him to carry on coughing. If, however, he becomes weak or cannot cough any more, bend him gently forwards and give five slaps between the shoulder blades. Stop if the object comes out or appears in the mouth. It is important to remember that these slaps should be quite firm as your aim is to dislodge the object. After five slaps, check in the person's mouth to see if the object has become dislodged.

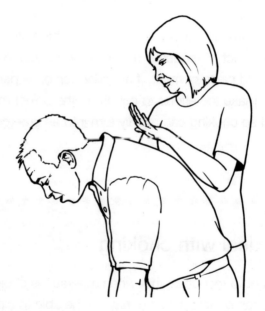

Fig 12 How to give back slaps

If back slaps fail to dislodge the object you must carry out abdominal thrusts.

> **one-minute** *wonder*
>
> **Q** Should I put my fingers into a person's mouth to remove
> something if he is choking?
> **A** Only if you can see the object. Never put your finger blindly
> into a person's mouth or perform a sweep with your fingers.

⑤ ● ⑤

abdominal thrusts

You may be familiar with this procedure as it was previously
known – the 'Heimlich Manoeuvre'. Your aim, when carrying out
treatment, is to dislodge the object by pushing the air from the
lungs up the windpipe, so it will force the object up into the
mouth.

To do abdominal thrusts, stand behind the person and put both
arms around the upper part of the abdomen between the navel
and the bottom of the breastbone. Make a fist with your hands
and pull sharply upwards and inwards five times. Stop if the
object pops out or appears in the mouth. If the person is very
frail reduce the force you use to do the thrusts whilst still
exerting enough force to remove the object.

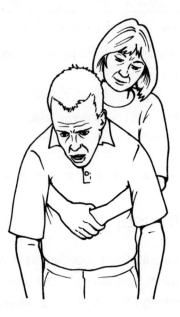

Fig 13 How to do abdominal thrusts

Either the back slaps or the abdominal thrusts will usually be successful and very often the first back slap is enough to move the object and allow it to come out.

If, however, the first efforts fail, carry out up to five back slaps and up to five abdominal thrusts three times and then call for an ambulance.

If at any time the blockage of the airway is sufficient to cause the older person to stop breathing and subsequently lose consciousness you will need to resuscitate him (see Chapter 2).

You should give rescue breaths making five attempts to give two effective rescue breaths. If successful, the chest will rise as you blow into the mouth and the person will get some oxygen into the lungs. If not successful you should give 15 chest compressions in an attempt to dislodge the object. You should alternate two rescue breath attempts and 15 chest compressions until the emergency services arrive and take over from you.

 key skills

To treat a person who is choking, you should firstly encourage him to cough. If he cannot move the object, give up to five back slaps between the shoulder blades. If back slaps don't work, you should do abdominal thrusts – carry out up to five of these. If this has not worked you should repeat back slaps and chest thrusts three times then call for an ambulance.

one-minute wonder

Q You say you should have five attempts to get two breaths into the person if he collapses. Why this many?

A By blowing into the person's mouth you might be able to dislodge the object by the pressure of your breath. This may mean the blockage will end up in the lung, but it will ensure the person will be able to breathe again.

one-minute wonder

Q Is there risk of doing any damage as a result of doing chest compressions on a person who has choked and is unconscious?

A A person who is unconscious as a result of a choking incident is in a critical condition. By doing chest compressions you are trying to dislodge the object. This procedure is not without risk, but these actions are in the patient's interest and take priority over risk of damage.

summary

Choking can be embarrassing and the immediate response of the person choking is to try and stifle it to hide their embarrassment. Back slaps delivered with sufficient force usually resolve the problem. If they don't, combine back slaps with abdominal thrusts and if the person goes unconscious, attempt rescue breaths and carry out chest compressions.

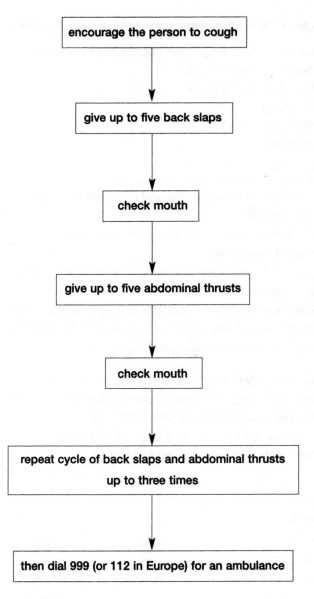

How to treat choking

self-testers ▬▬▬▬▬▬▬▬▬▬▬▬▬▬▬▬▬▬▬▬▬▬▬

1 Which of the following signs should you look out for if you suspect a person is choking?
   a difficulty breathing and clutching the throat
   b coughing
   c having a seizure
   d screaming

2 To do abdominal thrusts you should:
   a stand behind the person and put both arms on his breastbone
   b make a fist with your hands and pull sharply upwards and inwards five times
   c make a fist with your hands and pull sharply upwards and downwards five times
   d stand behind the person and put both arms around the upper part of the abdomen between the naval and the bottom of the breastbone

3 To treat a person who is choking you should deliver a cycle of
   a five back slaps and five abdominal thrusts
   b five back slaps and six abdominal thrusts
   c three back slaps and five abdominal thrusts
   d one back slap and one abdominal thrust

answers
1 **a** and **b**
2 **b** and **d**
3 **a**

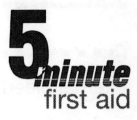
first aid

4

bleeding

One of the key functions of blood is to carry oxygen around the body, in particular to the vital organs including the heart, brain and kidneys. Any significant reduction in the amount of blood in the body can be life threatening. There are two main types of bleeding: internal and external. External bleeding is easier to diagnose because it is visible and the treatment is much more straightforward than for internal bleeding. Talking about blood and bleeding is off-putting for many people, as is seeing it. However, injuries resulting in blood loss remain among the most common first-aid situations you are likely to encounter. While the sight of blood is unpleasant for many people, there are only a very small number who will actually faint at the sight of it. Your wish to become involved and treat the person will probably overtake your fear of blood.

Ⓢ • Ⓢ

internal bleeding

It can be very difficult to diagnose internal bleeding. Nevertheless, the things you should consider if you suspect this type of bleeding are:

- the history of the incident
- what has happened
- has something fallen on to the person?
- has the person fallen onto something or has there been an impact (in particular to the abdomen)?

The abdominal area is particularly vulnerable in the case of an impact and, as the abdomen houses many of the body's key organs such as the liver and spleen, it is particularly susceptible to internal bleeding with life-threatening implications if not diagnosed. If you suspect internal bleeding, look at the area. Take into account the history of what has happened. Does the person appear to be going into shock? If so, is this disproportionate to the injuries you can see? Is he breathing more rapidly? Is his pulse rate increasing? Is there evidence of bruising and is the area tender? You also need to remember that blood may be visible. As mentioned, the blood loss you see externally may be disproportionate to the shock the injured person is experiencing.

For the treatment of internal bleeding, lay the person down and raise his legs. Loosen any tight clothing, especially around the abdomen, and get help as early as possible. Continue to monitor the person until the ambulance arrives (see page 61 on shock).

⑤ ● ⑤

external bleeding

As the term implies, external bleeding refers to blood lost outside the body, usually in the form of a serious wound. The severity of a wound depends on its location, its size and its depth. Severe blood loss occurs when there is damage to the large blood vessels that lie beneath the skin. The two most common types of blood vessels are veins and arteries. Arteries are the tubes that carry the blood, which is rich in oxygen, away from the heart. Veins return the blood back to the heart.

Any wound that involves damage to the arteries or veins can result in a serious loss of blood. Severe blood loss will result in the injured person looking pale, and the skin will be cold and clammy to touch. The person may appear confused, be yawning or ultimately, may fall unconscious.

severe bleeding

Your aim when treating a severe bleed is to stop the bleeding as quickly as possible and to minimize the risk of infection.

To treat a severe bleed, you should first expose the wound by cutting away any clothing. Then apply direct pressure over the

wound, ideally with a pad. You or the injured person can do this.
Once you have applied pressure, you should raise the injured
area above the level of the heart if possible. Help the person to
sit down or, preferably, to lie on the ground, and if a limb is
affected, keep the injured limb elevated. Tie the dressing in place
with a bandage. It is important to keep the injured part raised,
and if it is the arm that is bleeding, this can be done with a sling.
Once this treatment has been applied, call for an ambulance.

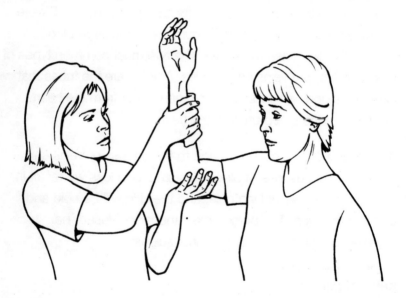

Fig 14 Raising and supporting an injured limb

Continue to check the blood circulation beyond the bandage by
pressing the nail of the finger or toe. If the circulation is good,

the nail bed will turn white when pressed and normal colour will return within a few seconds after release. If normal colour does not return, it probably means you have bandaged the limb too tightly. Release the bandage immediately and reapply it a little less tightly.

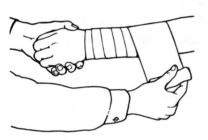
(a) Apply a dressing

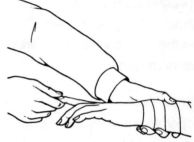
(b) Press the nail to check if the dressing is too tight

Fig 15 How to apply a dressing

---

one-minute wonder

Q I learnt in my first-aid course many years ago that you should apply a tourniquet to your arm if you cut it badly. Is this true?

A Tourniquets were once widely used for treating bleeding. However, this is no longer an approved first-aid procedure because it may cause reduced blood supply to the whole arm when the aim is only to stop the blood from the actual wound.

Older people are more vulnerable to serious wounds for two reasons. First, their blood vessels become more fragile and easier to damage. Second, the skin layers become thinner as we get older. This does not only results in wrinkles; in first-aid terms, it makes it easier to damage the skin.

One of the most common life-threatening injuries that can happen to older people is damage to a varicose vein which results in a severe bleed. This condition, which usually develops in the legs, can result in serious blood loss if the vein is knocked or damaged.

In the case of varicose veins the valves in the veins no longer operate efficiently so blood collects in the veins and this results in a stretching of the veins. Hence the wobbly appearance of the veins on the surface of the skin. This means that the injured person can lose a significant amount of blood in a short period of time.

To treat this type of bleeding, you should lay the person on the ground on his back, raising the injured leg as high as possible. You can kneel down and support his leg on your shoulders if necessary. Apply direct pressure on the wound with your hands (wear gloves if available), ideally over a pad. Maintain the pressure until the bleeding has slowed down. Bandage the pad in place. Check for signs of circulation as described in Chapter 2 on page 39. Call for an ambulance. Keep the leg elevated until the ambulance arrives.

key skills

To treat a wound resulting in severe blood loss, you should remove any clothing from around the wound. Apply direct pressure to the wound using your hands or ideally a pad. Call for an ambulance and reassure the person.

one-minute wonder

Q Throughout the chapter, you refer to significant blood loss. What does this mean in terms of blood loss from the body?

A The average person has about 5 litres (8 pints) of blood in his body. It is possible to lose up to 20 per cent of your blood volume before the situation becomes significant and shock starts to develop.

⑤ ● ⑤

shock

There are many causes of shock, including bleeding, burns, severe vomiting and diarrhoea. In fact, anything that results in the decreased volume of fluid in the body can cause shock.

It is important at this point to highlight the difference between clinical shock, the kind we are dealing with here, and shock which is an emotional response to something seen or heard. We often hear people say 'I'm in shock', possibly as a result of hearing some bad news or some good news; it is almost misleading to call this shock as this tends to be a temporary emotional response. Clinical shock is the body's physical response to a condition or injury and it can be life threatening unless it is treated properly.

If a person is going into shock, you will probably notice that the pulse rate increases and the skin looks pale. Keep observing the person's face for any change in colour. If you touch the skin it will feel cold and damp; we often refer to this as clammy skin. The person may complain of feeling thirsty, but also feeling sick. This often results in the person retching or bringing up small amounts of vomit. As shock progresses, the signs and symptoms tend to change. The person may develop cyanosis, which is the term used to describe the bluish tinge that appears around the lips and ear lobes. The person may also complain of feeling giddy, he may have difficulty focusing upon his surroundings, and appear increasingly weak. You may also notice that the breathing rate increases as the body tries to get enough oxygen into the lungs.

The treatment of shock varies depending on the cause. It is crucial, therefore, to treat the cause, and in this section we are looking at shock caused by bleeding. A person in shock should not be left on their own. Get someone else if possible and continue to talk to the person and reassure him while providing care. Avoid giving the person anything to eat or drink. Remember in serious cases of shock that the person may go unconscious, and subsequently be prepared to place him in the

recovery position (see Chapter 2, page 36) or resuscitate if
necessary (see Chapter 2, page 39).

To treat shock, lay the person down on his back to avoid any
unnecessary movement. Keep the person warm by using a
blanket or bystanders' excess clothing – fleeces are really good
for this purpose. A person in shock may feel cold on the hottest
day or in the warmest climate. Raise the legs above the level of
the heart; use a chair or anything available. If nothing is available,
ask a bystander to hold the person's legs in an elevated position
until you get something better to rest them on. This results in a
greater level of circulation in the body by moving the blood which
is in the legs to the key organs that require it such as the brain
and the heart. It is also important to keep reassuring the person.
Talk to him, keep him warm, and monitor him closely until the
ambulance arrives.

---

one-minute wonder

Q I was told that in a case of shock you should put clothing
under a person rather than over them. Is this true?

A A person can lose a lot of body heat if they are lying on
cold or wet ground. Ideally you should place a blanket or
clothing under and over the person. If you put something
under him it is best to put the blanket on the ground first to
avoid any unnecessary movement.

key skills

If a person is in shock, lay him down, raise his legs and keep him warm. Get someone to dial 999 (or 112 in Europe).

⑤ ● ⑤

crush injury

Older people very often spend time doing DIY projects in their retirement and so increase the risk of crush injuries. A crush injury may occur when a heavy object falls onto a person's abdomen or upper leg or onto their fingers and hands. If the DIY project is a big project large metal joists or masonry can fall on a person.

The most common injuries associated with crush injuries are fractures of the lower legs, pelvis or fingers. There is also the risk of internal bleeding and damage to the internal organs, which are located in the abdomen. The treatment for a crush injury very much depends on how long the individual has been crushed. Treatment will differ if the person is crushed for less than 15 minutes and if the person is crushed for more than 15 minutes.

less than 15 minutes

If the person is crushed for less than 15 minutes, it is important to remove the object that is causing the crushing as quickly as possible. Remember to put on gloves if they are available. Cover any external wound to minimize bleeding, check for any fractures, and treat the person for shock (see page 61). Call 999 for an ambulance. Continue to sit with the person and monitor his condition. Check his pulse and breathing and reassure him until the ambulance arrives. Watch for symptoms of shock.

more than 15 minutes

The treatment for an individual who is crushed for more than 15 minutes varies from that described above because of the risk of prolonged crushing. This can result in reduced blood supply and numbness below the point of the injury, which in turn starves the body tissues and muscles of adequate blood supply. As a result, there can be a build-up of toxic substances which, if released, can spread around the body possibly resulting in kidney failure. It is more commonly known in the medical world as the 'crush syndrome'. This is an extremely serious condition and can on occasions be fatal. Therefore, your aim when a person has been crushed for more than 15 minutes is not to release him or to remove the crushing object. Leave the object in place and call for an ambulance immediately. Give precise details of the accident, how it occurred and how long the person has been crushed. Continue to monitor the person and give him reassurance until the ambulance arrives.

key skills

If a person is crushed for less than 15 minutes, remove the crushing object as quickly as possible, treat any obvious wounds and fractures and monitor for internal bleeding and shock. Dial 999 (or 112 in Europe), and get the person to hospital as quickly as possible.

If a person has been crushed for more than 15 minutes, dial 999 (or 112 in Europe) for an ambulance immediately. Do not remove the object, but do treat any other obvious injury, and continue to reassure the person.

summary

Don't be put off by the sight of blood. Quickly inspect the wound, find where the blood is coming from, apply pressure and elevate the limb. Call for an ambulance if necessary. As with most first-aid practices it is important to reassure the person and give him some confidence in your ability. Remember, don't give him anything to eat or drink if he is going to be treated in hospital.

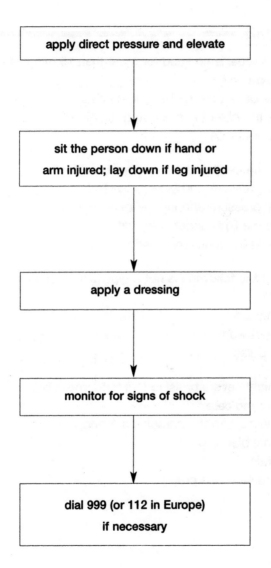

How to treat severe external bleeding

self-testers ▬▬▬▬▬▬▬▬▬▬▬▬▬▬▬▬▬▬▬▬▬

1 If an individual is crushed for more than 15 minutes what should you do?
   a lift the object off the body immediately
   b leave the object in place and dial 999 (or 112 in Europe) for an ambulance

2 What is the treatment for external bleeding?
   a apply pressure and elevate the limb
   b apply pressure and lay the person down
   c place the limb under cold water
   d place in the recovery position

3 Which of the following is not a typical sign of shock?
   a thirst
   b feeling sick
   c red and warm skin
   d slow pulse

4 What might severe bruising and tenderness of a person's abdomen indicate?
   a problems with the person's appendix
   b internal bleeding
   c a sprain
   d severe stomach cramp

answers
1 **b**
2 **a** and **b**
3 **c** and **d**
4 **b**

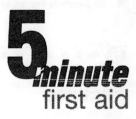
first aid

5

trips and falls

Falling is a common experience for older people. Evidence suggests that about 30 per cent of those aged 65 and over fall each year, rising to 50 per cent for those aged 80 or more. Rates of falling increase with rising rates of illness. Falls may be symptoms of underlying disease processes, impairments and disabilities but may also be the cause of disability. Factors that lead to falling include postural difficulties, declining vision, decreasing muscle power and reduced reaction times. The bone-thinning disease, osteoporosis, contributes to the incidence of fractures, especially in women.

The consequences of falling include sprains, strains and fractures. The most common fractures in the older person are of the wrist and hip.

⑤ • ⑤

fractures

facts about fractures

A fracture is a break in a bone. It is described as 'closed' when the skin around it is intact, and as 'open' if there is an accompanying wound or the broken bone end is protruding through the skin. A fracture is described as 'stable' when the broken bone ends do not move – either because they are not completely broken or because they are impacted. A fracture is described as 'unstable' when the bone ends can move around; they can then damage surrounding tissues such as blood vessels and nerves.

⑤ • ⑤

the wrist fracture

how would you recognize a fractured wrist?

A fractured wrist commonly happens when a person falls and puts out a hand to 'save himself'. The fracture site is painful and tender and the wrist will appear to be deformed, especially when compared to the uninjured wrist. The wrist joint is also frequently sprained and it may be difficult to decide whether the injury has resulted in a sprain or a fracture. You should suspect a fracture, and treat a painful wrist as a fracture until this has been excluded.

If you suspect a fracture, you should keep the wrist as still as possible. This can be done by asking the person to gently bend the arm at the elbow so that the arm is across the body and then it can be supported by the other arm. Surround the arm in soft padding such as a small towel or a thick layer of cotton wool. If you have a first-aid kit, it is best to place the arm in a sling for the journey to hospital.

how to put on an arm sling

To put on an arm sling you will need a triangular bandage and a safety pin. With the arm supported across the body, slide one end of the bandage through the hollow under the elbow. Pull the end across the body and around the back of the neck and place it in the hollow just above the collarbone on the side of the injury. Then bring the lower end of the bandage up over the arm so that it supports the injured arm. Pull the two ends together and tie a knot so that it rests in the hollow above the collarbone on the injured side. Tuck the ends under the knot and then fold any excess bandage that remains at the elbow and secure it with the safety pin. The arm is then supported and can rest on the chest. Take or send the person to hospital.

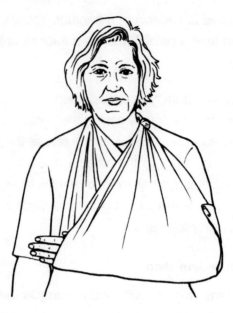

Fig 16 An arm sling

---

one-minute wonder

Q What can I do to improvise a sling if I don't have a first-aid
  kit?

A If the person is wearing a jacket or a cardigan, you can
  improvise by turning one side up over the arm and
  fastening it to the top of the garment with a safety pin.

⑤ • ⑤

the hip fracture

how would you recognize a fractured hip?

A fractured hip usually occurs when a person falls directly onto that side. The fracture involves the neck of the thigh bone or femur and is usually a stable fracture with the bone ends impacted together. This sometimes means that even though there is discomfort, the person can walk with this fracture for some time before the discomfort becomes difficult to tolerate and the fracture is discovered.

If there is a history of falling onto the hip, accompanied by discomfort around the site of the injury, especially when trying to walk, then you should suspect a fracture. There will also be a shortening of the affected leg and turning outwards of the knee and foot. This is best seen when the person is lying down.

If the person has a fractured hip, you should encourage him to lie down and arrange for him to go to hospital in an ambulance. Treat shock if present by insulating from the cold with blankets or clothing. Do not give the person anything to eat or drink because a general anaesthetic may be needed in hospital.

⑤ ● ⑤

the skull fracture

how would you recognize a skull fracture?

A skull fracture can result from a fall or a bang on the head. With a skull fracture there is a danger that the underlying brain will be damaged either by a piece of the skull itself or by bleeding into the brain. Always suspect a skull fracture when an injury to the head is accompanied by impaired consciousness. There may be a wound or bruise on the head, bruising around one or both eyes, and fluid or watery blood coming from the ear or the nose.

If you suspect a skull fracture, you should help the person to lie down and keep his head as still as possible. Don't turn the head in case there is also a neck injury. Dial 999 (or 112 in Europe) for an ambulance. If there is fluid coming from the nose or the ear, cover with a pad but do not try to plug it. Monitor and record the pulse, breathing and, importantly, the level of response.

The methods used to monitor the person's level of response are detailed in Chapter 2, page 35.

⑤ ● ⑤

rib fractures

how would you recognize fractured ribs?

Rib fractures are usually a result of falling onto the chest. The person usually complains of sharp pain at the site of the fracture, and pain when taking a deep breath. Sometimes several ribs are fractured leading to a 'flail chest', whch is when the broken ribs become detached from the rest of the chest wall. The detached segment moves in when the person breathes in, and out when the person breathes out. This is the reverse of normal breathing movements and will lead to breathing difficulty and shortness of breath.

If you suspect a fractured rib, you should support the arm on the injured side in an arm sling and arrange for the person to go to hospital.

---

one-minute *wonder*

Q Should I tape up the chest if I think ribs are broken?

A No. This action will prevent the person from breathing normally and may lead to underlying infection later.

---

⑤ ● ⑤

fractures of the spine

how would you recognize a fracture of the spine?

The bones of the spine are commonly affected by osteoporosis in older people and may therefore fracture easily on impact or as a result of a fall. There may only be a slight injury. In this situation, the bones usually collapse into one another and cause a stable fracture. The risk of damage to the spinal cord and nerves is less than it would be after a traumatic spinal fracture in a younger person.

The person will complain of severe pain in the back around the site of the fracture and there will be tenderness in the skin. It will be painful to walk, bend and twist the spine.

If you suspect a fractured spine, you should help the person to lie down. Reassure and advise him to stay as still as possible and make him comfortable by supporting him with pillows, rolled towels and blankets placed around the body. Keep the person still and comfortable until a medical assessment is made. If you suspect a fracture in the spine at the neck, support the head until a medical assessment is made.

how to support the head

Kneel behind the person's head after telling him what you are going to do. Take firm hold of the head, with your hands over the person's ears. Do not completely cover the ears, instead leave a gap between your fingers so that the person can hear you. Steady and support the head, trying not to move it. Try to keep the head, neck and back aligned so that you provide the least harmful position for someone with a suspected fracture of the spine in the neck. Make yourself comfortable so that you can maintain this support until help arrives.

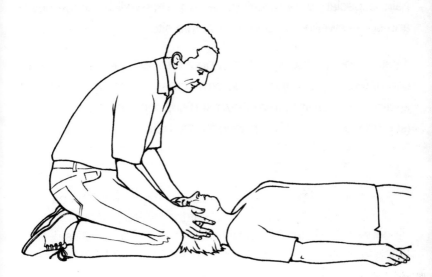

Fig 17 How to support the head

⑤ ● ⑤

fracture of the upper part of the arm

how would you recognize a fracture of the upper arm?

When the upper arm breaks in the older person, usually as a result of a fall onto the arm, it is common for the break to be at the upper end of the bone. The broken bone ends usually stay in place so it is a stable fracture, and for this reason the break may not be immediately apparent. There is, however, likely to be pain, especially when moving the arm. There will be tenderness and some swelling around the fracture site.

If you suspect a fracture of the upper arm, ask the person to sit down. Gently place the injured arm across the body and support it with the other arm. Immobilize and support the arm in a sling (see pages 71 and 72). Arrange for the person to go to hospital.

 key skills

If you suspect a person has a fracture, treat them on the basis that this is the case. Remember that the injured person's account or a bystander's description of what happened is important so that you can decide on the extent of the injury.

⑤ • ⑤

dislocations

A dislocation is a joint injury in which bones are partially or fully pulled out of normal position. In an older person who has arthritis with deformed joints it can be difficult to decide when dislocation has taken place. There is usually severe pain and unusual difficulty moving the joint. The joints commonly dislocated are the shoulder, jaw and the joints of the fingers and thumbs.

how would you recognize a dislocation?

You should suspect a dislocation if the person has severe pain and swelling of the joint, unusual difficulty moving the joint and, in some cases, may appear to have a joint deformity. If you suspect a dislocation, advise the person to keep the painful joint still. Support the painful joint in a position of greatest comfort. If the dislocation affects the shoulder or hand, immobilize and support the limb in a sling. If the jaw is dislocated, give the person a soft pad and hold this against the jaw for support and arrange for the person to go to hospital.

🌑 *key skills*

In the event of a dislocation, ask the injured person to stay in the position that is least painful. Immobilize using a sling. Take the person to hospital.

---

one-minute wonder

Q If I think a finger is dislocated can I put it back into place?

A It is best not to try this as there may be a fracture accompanying the dislocation and you may do more damage. Also, pulling a joint that is dislocated is very painful.

Ⓢ • Ⓢ

sprains and strains

The ankle is the most commonly sprained joint, and the injury very often results from falling off a roadside kerb and twisting the ankle. All sprains and strains are characterized by pain, tenderness, and swelling and bruising around the site of the injury. It is often difficult to tell the difference between a sprain and a fracture. If there is a lot of pain, it is always best to assume it is a fracture and have a medical assessment to rule it out.

If you suspect a sprain or a strain, you should use the RICE procedure:

R Rest the injured site
I Apply ice or a cold compress
C Compress the injury
E Elevate the injured limb.

---

one-minute *wonder*

Q What is the difference between a sprain and a strain?

A A sprain is a result of an overstretching of the ligaments that support a joint. A strain is a 'pulled' muscle when the muscle is stretched or partially torn.

how to apply ice to the site of an injury

Partially fill a plastic bag with small ice cubes, or use a bag of frozen peas. Wrap the bag in a dry cloth and hold it on the injury for ten minutes, replacing the pack as needed. Do not apply ice directly onto the skin, as it will lead to a cold burn.

After cooling with ice, apply comfortable and even compression to the site of the injury by surrounding the area with a thick layer of padding such as cotton wool. Secure the padding with a roller bandage.

how to apply a roller bandage

Position yourself in front of the person on the injured side. Keep the site of the injury well supported while you are applying the bandage. Place the tail (the rolled part of the bandage is called the head and the unrolled part the tail) of the bandage below the injury and, working from the inside of the limb outwards, make two straight turns to anchor the tail in place. Then make a spiral of turns and work up the limb. Finish with one straight turn and secure the bandage with a safety pin.

After applying a roller bandage it is important to make sure it is not too tight around the limb and that it is not 'cutting off' the circulation. Always ask if it is too tight and check the circulation below the bandage.

If the pain is severe or the person is unable to use the injured limb, arrange for assessment in hospital. Otherwise advise the person to rest and, if the pain persists, ask for medical assessment.

 key skills

A sprain or a strain should be treated using RICE.

---

one-minute *wonder*

Q   Is it true that a sprain or a strain is more painful than a fracture?

A   It can be, but this often depends on the site and severity of the injury as well as the pain threshold of the injured person. We certainly do not advise you to use the level of pain as an indication of whether it's a fracture or a strain or sprain.

---

summary

It is very difficult for a non-professional to differentiate between a sprain, strain, dislocation or fracture. Always treat the person on the basis that they have the worst injury. Remember the RICE acronym if you are treating a sprain or a strain.

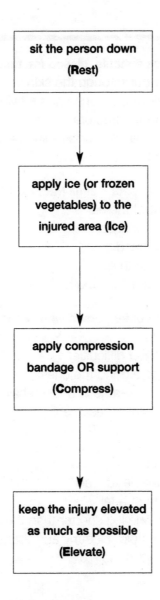

How to treat a sprain or strain (RICE)

self-testers ▬▬▬▬▬▬▬▬▬▬▬▬▬▬▬▬▬▬▬▬▬▬▬▬

1 What features does a stable, closed fracture have?
   a the bone sticks out through the skin
   b there is little risk of the bone ends moving around
   c a wound around the fracture
   d a high risk of damaging surrounding nerves
   e intact skin over the fracture site

2 You must always suspect a skull fracture if there is:
   a fluid coming out of the ear
   b impaired consciousness
   c a wound on the head
   d bruising around both eyes
   e an inability to open the mouth

3 When managing an older person with suspected fractured ribs, what should you do?
   a watch for breathing difficulties
   b apply a bandage around the chest
   c tell the person to breathe in a fast, shallow manner
   d arrange for medical assessment
   e tell the person to lie on his back for sleeping

4 How is a fracture of the hip recognized?
   a the person is unable to walk
   b there is a history of a fall
   c the person has one leg shorter than the other
   d the person feels cold, clammy and dizzy
   e there is pain around the hip

5 If a person has a head injury what should you suspect?
  a an accompanying neck injury
  b a change in the level of consciousness
  c a discharge of blood from the mouth
  d a fracture of the skull
  e a heart attack

1 When treating a sprain or a strain, what do the letters RICE mean?

  R_____

  I_____

  C_____

  E_____

answers
1 **b** and **e**
2 **a**, **b**, **c** and **d**
3 **a** and **d**
4 **a**, **b**, **c**, **d** and **e**
5 **a**, **b** and **d**
6 Rest, Ice, Compression, Elevation

what has happened. You should then dial 999 (or 112 in
Europe) for an ambulance, or ask someone else to do this for
you.

Help the person to lie down with his head and shoulders
supported, or if the person is already in bed make sure that he
remains there. You should also loosen any restricting clothing
and ensure that the sufferer is not given anything to eat or drink
because there is a danger he may choke. If one side of the face
is droopy, use a small towel to soak up any dribble and, if
possible, monitor and record the pulse, breathing and level of
response regularly until help arrives.

---

one-minute wonder

Q Can I wait until the following day to send a person to
hospital who has had a stroke?

A No. The stroke victim will benefit from early admission and,
if the stroke is the result of a blood clot, drugs can be given
to try to dissolve the clot.

---

 key skills

Sudden loss of movement of the limbs on one side, or the
feeling that one side of the face is paralysed can indicate that
the person has had a stroke.

The main risk associated with a heart attack is that the heart will stop beating and the attack will be fatal. This is known as cardiac arrest. Therefore, early recognition and admission to hospital are vital.

---

one-minute wonder

Q If a person I know has heart disease and complains of sudden indigestion can I assume it is indigestion?

A No. You must always suspect a heart attack and dial 999 (or 112 in Europe) for an ambulance.

---

how would you recognize a heart attack?

If a person is suffering from persistent cramp-like pain in the chest, or pain that spreads to the jaw, arms and/or through to the back, and is experiencing either shortness of breath, dizziness, nausea, sweating and has an ashen colour of the skin, suspect that there is something seriously wrong. A rapid and possibly irregular pulse is a further sign of a possible heart attack.

If you suspect a heart attack, make the person as comfortable as possible to ease the strain on the heart. Leaning back against some support with the knees bent is often the most comfortable position. Call for an ambulance and make sure that you say that you suspect a heart attack.

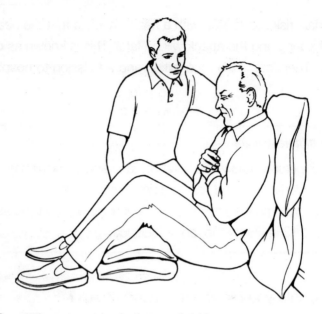

Fig 19 Support the person and make them comfortable

If you can be confident that the person has no allergy to aspirin, ask him to slowly chew a 300 mg aspirin tablet. If the person has any angina medication, encourage him to take it. Whilst you are waiting for the ambulance, monitor and record the person's pulse, breathing and level of response. Remember that if the person suddenly loses consciousness you should proceed as illustrated in Chapter 2.

key skills

If you suspect a heart attack call for an ambulance, give the person an aspirin, make him comfortable and continue to reassure him while you are waiting for the ambulance. Check if the person is on any medication and advise the ambulance crew of this.

---

one-minute *wonder*

Q I'm still confused about how I, as a member of the public, would know the difference between a case of angina and a heart attack.

A A person who has angina will probably know he has the condition; he may have experienced similar episodes, and the pain will ease with rest. A heart-attack victim may never have experienced this before, and the pain does not get better with rest. However, if you are in doubt you should call for an ambulance.

---

one-minute *wonder*

Q Is it safe to give aspirin to someone I think is having a heart attack?

A No drug administration can ever be absolutely safe but clinical evidence shows that the benefits of the aspirin outweigh the risks if the aspirin is chewed slowly and the person is not allergic to it.

⑤ • ⑤

seizures

A seizure is a term used to describe sudden involuntary contractions in many muscles in the body caused by abnormal electrical activity in the brain. A seizure is otherwise known as a fit or a convulsion, and the most common cause is epilepsy. However, seizures can also take place as a result of a head injury, shortage of oxygen or glucose in the brain, and some poisons including the consumption of excess alcohol.

how would you recognize a seizure?

Very often a seizure follows a pattern. This pattern begins before the muscle contractions even start with the person saying that he is experiencing an abnormality of one of the senses such as sight or smell. This is called an 'aura' and heralds the onset of the seizure. The person will then suddenly lose consciousness and his body will become rigid.

Shaking movements follow and the jaw will become clenched, breathing will stop and sometimes the person bites his tongue. There may also be a loss of control of the bladder and the bowel resulting in incontinence.

After the shaking, the muscles relax and consciousness returns but the person may feel frightened, dazed and confused and want to sleep.

If you witness a seizure, it is important that you take the correct action to ensure the best care of the person. It is vital that you do not try to interfere with the pattern of the seizure, but instead protect the person from injury by removing from the scene items such as hot liquids or sharp objects. If you can, place soft padding under the head to protect it.

When the seizure is over, give lots of reassurance and try to calm the person, allowing him to sleep if he wants. However, if the person remains unconscious, you must open the airway and, if breathing, place the person in the recovery position and call for an ambulance. Calling for an ambulance is particularly important if:

- the seizure continues for more than five minutes
- this is the person's first seizure
- one seizure closely follows another
- the person sustains other injuries that require urgent medical treatment.

You should also regularly monitor and record the person's pulse, breathing and level of response until help arrives.

> **one-minute** *wonder*
>
> **Q** I was told that if a person is having a seizure I should put
> something in the mouth. Is this correct?
>
> **A** No, there is no need to place anything in the mouth of a
> person during a seizure. If you attempt this you may cause
> damage to the person's mouth or you may get injured.

⑤ ● ⑤

problems with diabetic control

Diabetes is a chronic medical condition in which the body fails to
produce sufficient amounts of the hormone insulin. Normally insulin
is produced in the pancreas and its role is to control the sugar
metabolism in the body. When there is a disturbance of the sugar
level in the blood a person may suffer from either hypoglycaemia
or hyperglycaemia. Hypoglycaemia means there is low blood
sugar and hyperglycaemia means there is high blood sugar.

types of diabetes

There are two types of diabetes: Type 1 and Type 2. In Type 1
diabetes there is an immune-related destruction of the insulin-
producing cells in the pancreas. This results in too little insulin in
the body and so hyperglycaemia occurs. It can happen in any
age group but is more common in younger people. Injected
insulin is used to control this type of diabetes.

Type 2 diabetes is the most common form and it accounts for around 90 per cent of all cases of diabetes. It usually occurs in older people. Its onset is gradual and it is associated with obesity, inactivity, and any evidence of the disease in the family's medical history. There is also some medical research that supports the idea that particular ethnic groups are more susceptible to diabetes. Diet, exercise and oral medication can usually control the hyperglycaemia.

With both types of diabetes, disturbances of control can occur which may result in either hypoglycaemia or hyperglycaemia.

how would you recognize hypoglycaemia?

At the start of all hypoglycaemic attacks a person may experience warning signs that he recognizes and therefore may be able to alert you to the 'hypo' starting.

Symptoms that may be apparent include:

- a history of missed meals or undertaking strenuous exercise that had not been planned or taken account of when eating and drinking
- the person wearing a warning bracelet or talisman
- hunger
- weakness
- feeling faint
- muscle tremors
- sweating

- cold, clammy skin
- a rapid pulse
- a rapid deterioration in responsiveness.

You should be aware that hypoglycaemia often has a very quick onset of symptoms.

If you suspect a person is having a hypoglycaemic attack and he is conscious, you should help him to sit down and rest, and give him a sugary drink or sweet food. Alternatively, if the person has glucose gel, help him to take it. However, if the person is not fully conscious you should not give him anything to eat or drink. Instead, open the airway and, if breathing, place in the recovery position and call for an ambulance.

 key skills

If you suspect a person is having a hypoglycaemic attack and he is conscious, give him a sugary drink or glucose gel. If he falls unconscious, place him in the recovery position.

one-minute wonder

Q Why do I give sugar to a person I think is hypoglycaemic?

A To raise the blood sugar as quickly as possible and stop the person from losing consciousness.

how would you recognize hyperglycaemia?

Hyperglycaemia is more difficult to recognize than hypoglycaemia. If the person is a known diabetic then you should be more aware that he could be experiencing hyperglycaemia. It often occurs with another illness such as a chest infection. The person may have warm, dry skin, a fruity sweet breath odour, and suffer from drowsiness and then loss of consciousness.

If you suspect hyperglycaemia, you should call for an ambulance and, if the person is drowsy or unconscious, you should place him in the recovery position. It is important to remember that while waiting for an ambulance to arrive you should regularly monitor and record the person's pulse, breathing and level of response.

---

one-minute *wonder*

Q If a person I know is diabetic but I don't know whether the problem is hypoglycaemia or hyperglycaemia will I do harm if I give sugar?

A To give sugar is good management as you will rapidly correct hypoglycaemia and do little harm if the problem is hyperglycaemia.

summary

As we become older our bodies become more susceptible to disease and illness. Many of these conditions are chronic in nature and do not interfere with people carrying on life as usual. However, despite our best efforts to manage these conditions it is inevitable that sometimes conditions enter an acute phase that require first aid. Many people lead full lives with these conditions and have a very good understanding of the condition, and so it is really important that you listen to their views about how they feel.

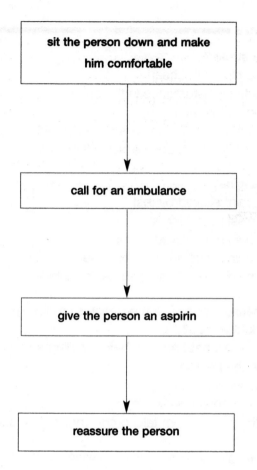

What to do if you suspect a heart attack

self-testers ▬▬▬▬▬▬▬▬▬▬▬▬▬▬▬▬▬▬

1 **What is a stroke?**
   a a blood clot in the heart
   b an electrical disturbance in the brain
   c a blood clot in the brain
   d a leakage from a blood vessel in the brain
   e a leakage from a blood vessel in the chest

2 **What is angina?**
   a chest pain relieved by rest
   b abdominal pain relieved by rest
   c chest pain not relieved by rest
   d chest pain brought on by exercise
   e chest pain relieved using an aerosol inhaler

3 **When treating a person you suspect is having a heart attack what should you do?**
   a wait to see what happens before calling an ambulance
   b ensure the person rests
   c give aspirin to swallow
   d make the person lie down
   e stop the person from taking any angina medication

4 **When managing a person who is having a seizure what should you do?**
   a try to open the airway
   b move the person to one side
   c try to restrain the person using force
   d remove any potential hazards
   e monitor the person closely after the seizure

5 **Signs of hypoglycaemia include:**
  a hunger
  b cold, clammy skin
  c rapid pulse rate
  d feeling faint
  e muscle tremors

answers
1 **c** and **d**
2 **a**, **d** and **e**
3 **b**
4 **d** and **e**
5 **a**, **b**, **c**, **d** and **e**

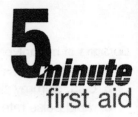

7

the use of common medicines, and drug poisoning

Advances in the development of medications have played a major part in improving the quality and extending the life of many people in our society. Many older people rely on tablets and other medication to maintain their well-being. You should remember that the effectiveness of this medication is dependent on the person taking it as prescribed.

Older people should exercise caution when taking medicines. This is due in part to the effects that medicines have on the body as age advances, and in part because older people may be unable to manage the medicines properly. They may also be taking a number of medicines for chronic conditions such as heart disease or diabetes and so the potential for error is high.

The role of first aid in this situation is not to advise on the medicines themselves but to be aware of medicines the older person may be taking and the risks associated with these. Particularly important in the caring situation is an awareness of the routine needed to manage the taking of the medicines.

---

one-minute wonder

Q If an older person is taking a number of medicines, is the chance of a bad reaction higher?

A Yes, older people are more sensitive to the effects of medicines, so the risk is higher.

---

tips for using medicines

Make sure the person has all the information necessary for the correct use of the medicine. Whenever possible, capsules and tablets should be taken standing up or in an upright sitting position. Capsules and tablets should be taken with water. If giving someone a liquid medicine, take care to measure it properly. When giving liquid medicines, shake the bottle before measuring out the dose. Hide the unpleasant taste of a medicine by giving the person a drink of cold water immediately after the medicine. Use medicines with a memory aid. If the person is taking more than one medicine, use a pill box with a strip for each day and individual compartments for different times of the day.

***one-minute* wonder**

Q Why is it important to take medicines standing or sitting upright and with water?

A Because if they are taken when lying down or without enough water the medicine might become stuck in the oesophagus. This can delay the action of the medicine and may damage the oesophagus.

---

⑤ ● ⑤

aspirin

Aspirin is a commonly used medicine, especially when given in low doses to help to prevent blood clots. It is used particularly if the person has heart disease such as angina, and it helps to reduce the incidence of heart attacks and strokes. (It is taken once daily for the prevention of blood clots.)

Aspirin is also used for the relief of pain, fever, and joint and muscle aches. It is present in many proprietary preparations sold over the counter, and it is taken for the relief of coughs and colds.

Aspirin should be taken every four to six hours as necessary with or after milk or food for the relief of pain or fever.

adverse effects

Adverse effects are more likely to occur with high doses, and can be reduced by taking the aspirin with food or by using the enteric-coated tablets. The most common effect is indigestion and less likely effects are:

- rash
- nausea breathlessness/wheezing
- ringing in the ears and dizziness
- blood in the vomit or black faeces.

overdose

The signs of an overdose are:

- restlessness
- stomach pain
- blurred vision
- vomiting
- severe ringing in the ears.

In the case of an overdose, seek urgent medical help.

---

one-minute *wonder*

Q What does it mean if someone has black faeces?

A It means there is bleeding somewhere in the bowel, and the blood looks black when mixed with the faeces. This is a serious sign and an urgent medical assessment is needed.

Ⓢ • Ⓢ

beta-blockers

This is a large group of medicines that includes all those whose spellings end in 'olol', such as Atenolol, Metoprolol, Propranolol and Bisoprolol. They are used in the management of irregular heart rhythms, angina and high blood pressure, and may also be used to reduce anxiety.

Most are taken once or twice a day. A missed dose should be taken as soon as possible, and sudden withdrawal may lead to dangerous worsening of the underlying medical problem.

adverse effects

The adverse effects are usually temporary and diminish with long-term use. The most common are:
- muscle aches
- dry eyes.

Less likely are:
- a headache
- a rash
- nightmares/sleeplessness
- breathing difficulties
- dizziness.

overdose

Overdosing is rare but occasionally breathing difficultues can occur. In the case of an overdose, report the symptoms to a doctor.

one-minute *wonder*

Q I have heard that sometimes actors and musicians take
  beta-blockers before a performance, is this true?

A Yes, they do so to relieve their anxiety and calm their nerves.

digoxin

Digoxin is used in the treatment of heart failure and some heart
rhythm abnormalities. It acts by increasing the force of the
heartbeat, making it more effective in pumping blood around the
body. Digoxin is taken up to three times daily.

adverse effects

Adverse effects include:
- tiredness
- nausea
- loss of appetite.

Less likely are:
- confusion
- visual disturbance
- palpitations.

overdose

An overdose leads to:

- severe weakness
- palpitations
- chest pain
- loss of consciousness.

In the case of an overdose, seek urgent medical help in all cases. If unconscious, place the person in the recovery position (see page 36).

⑤ ● ⑤

diuretics

Diuretic medicines act on the kidneys to help the body turn excess body water into urine. This means that body tissues become less waterlogged and the heart can then work more efficiently. Diuretics are used to treat high blood pressure, heart failure and some kidney disorders. There are many diuretics available but the two most common ones are Furosemide and Bendroflumethiazide. Furosemide is taken once daily. Bendroflumethiazide is taken daily or on alternate days.

adverse effects

Adverse effects are rare, but include:

- dizziness and nausea.

Less likely are:
- lethargy
- palpitations
- muscle pains
- a rash.

overdose

An overdose is unlikely to have any serious effects.

⑤ • ⑤

statins

Statins is a group of cholesterol-lowering medicines. Simvastatin is one of these medicines and has been in use since 1989. These drugs block the manufacture of cholesterol in the liver and, as a result, the blood levels of cholesterol fall. The medicines are used in people who have high levels of cholesterol in the blood and who are at risk of developing, or already have, heart disease. The medicine is taken once a day at night.

adverse effects

Adverse effects are rare. Occasionally the following can occur:
- abdominal pain
- a skin rash
- nausea
- constipation
- muscle pain and weakness.

overdose

An overdose is rare but large overdoses can lead to liver problems.

In the case of an overdose, tell a doctor.

⑤ • ⑤

vasodilators

Vasodilators are medicines that widen blood vessels, usually by relaxing the muscle around the blood vessels. They are used mainly to treat high blood pressure and angina. They include a large number of medicines such as:

- ACE inhibitors – all those that end in 'pril', such as Captopril
- Calcium channel blockers such as Amlodipine and Nifedipine
- Nitrates – Glyceryl trinitrate (GTN), Mononitrate

captopril

This is started as a low dose and gradually increased to the correct level for the individual. A missed dose should be taken as soon as possible and the medicine should not be stopped without consulting a doctor.

adverse effects

Adverse effects include:
- a loss of taste
- a rash and cough.

Less likely are:
- a sore mouth
- dizziness and a sore throat
- swelling of the mouth and lips.

overdose

An overdose is rare but a large overdose may cause dizziness or fainting.

In the case of an overdose, tell a doctor.

amlodipine

Amlodipine is started as a low dose and gradually increased to the correct level for the individual. A missed dose should be taken as soon as possible and the medicine should not be stopped without consulting a doctor.

adverse effects

Adverse effects include:
- drowsiness
- sweating
- dry mouth
- constipation.

Less likely are:
- a sore throat
- difficulty passing urine
- palpitations.

overdose

An overdose will bring on palpitations and loss of consciousness. If unconscious, place the person in the recovery position (see page 36). Dial 999 for an ambulance.

glyceryl trinitrate (GTN)

GTN is one of the oldest medicines still in regular use. It is available in short-acting forms such as sublingual or buccal tablets or spray, and in long-acting forms such as slow release tablets and skin patches. It is used for the management of angina.

GTN can be taken in preventative doses three times daily as tablets; once daily as a patch; and every three hours as ointment. It can also be used as tablets or spray for relief at the onset of an angina attack or before exercise.

adverse effects

Adverse effects include:
- headache
- flushing
- dizziness.

overdose

A large overdose may lead to:
- dizziness
- vomiting

- a headache
- loss of consciousness.

In the case of an overdose, notify a doctor but seek urgent medical help if consciousness is lost. If unconscious, place the person in the recovery position (see page 36).

⑤ • ⑤

warfarin

Warfarin is an anticoagulant drug used to treat and prevent blood clots. It is used especially for people who have heart rhythm irregularities, previous strokes and heart valve replacements. It requires regular monitoring to ensure the maintenance dose is correct. Warfarin is taken once a day at the same time each day.

adverse effects

Adverse effects include:
- bleeding
- bruising
- dark faeces
- dark urine or bleeding.

These should be reported immediately.

Less likely are:
- fever
- nausea
- a rash
- hair loss
- jaundice
- abdominal pain.

overdose

The sign of an overdose is severe bleeding leading to loss of consciousness.

In the case of overdose, seek urgent medical help. Take measures to try to stop the bleeding. If the person is unconscious, place him in the recovery position.

---

one-minute wonder

Q I have heard that Warfarin doesn't mix with a lot of other drugs. Is this true?

A Yes, there is a large number of drugs that can react with Warfarin and increase the time for the blood to clot. This increases the chance of bleeding and so no other medicines must be taken without the approval of the doctor or pharmacist.

---

⑤ • ⑤

medicines used for diabetic control

insulin

Insulin is a hormone normally produced by the pancreas in the body and it acts to control blood sugar. In diabetes this hormone is absent or reduced, and synthetic insulin is needed to control the blood sugar. Insulin is used in all Type 1 diabetics and some Type 2 diabetics. It is given by injection and tailored to individual needs.

adverse effects

Adverse effects are rare.

overdose

An overdose will lead to hypoglycaemia, which needs immediate medical intervention (see page 97).

antidiabetic tablets

There are several medicines in this category. All act by encouraging the pancreas to produce insulin, and so can only be used when there is some pancreatic function. These medicines include Glibenclamide, Metformin and Tolbutamide.

Antidiabetic tablets are usually taken once a day but are tailored to individual needs and combined with diet.

adverse effects

Adverse effects include:
- weakness
- tremors
- sweating.

Less likely are:

- nausea
- rash
- jaundice.

overdose

An overdose will lead to hypoglycaemia.

In the case of an overdose, seek urgent medical help (see Chapter 6, page 97).

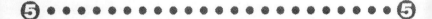

drug poisoning

If you suspect drug poisoning as a result of a drug overdose, it is important to take urgent action. This is particularly crucial if the person is:

- vomiting
- drowsy or unconscious
- breathing noisily or the breathing is shallow and laboured
- not breathing
- having a seizure.

Act as you would when dealing with an emergency (see Chapter 1, page 2). You may need to resuscitate (see Chapter 2) or deal with a seizure (see Chapter 6, page 94).

In addition, collect any evidence that will assist with the diagnosis such as empty containers, any medicines that remain with their containers, and vomited material.

summary

Medications should only be taken as prescribed. Medications that are out of date or are prescribed for someone else should not be taken. If you have any concerns about the medication being taken consult a doctor.

self-testers

1 What measures help an older person to take medication?
   a the use of a pill box
   b having the medicine in liquid form if possible
   c giving the medicine with a drink of alcohol
   d sitting upright when taking tablets
   e giving the person the correct information for the use of the medicine

2 What is aspirin used for?
   a to prevent blood clot formation
   b to relieve pain and fever
   c to reduce the incidence of stroke
   d to treat an infection in the urine
   e to treat stomach ulcers

3 **What are the effects of an overdose of aspirin?**
   a shortness of breath
   b ringing in the ears
   c blurred vision
   d pain when passing urine
   e abdominal pain

4 **Beta-blockers are used for the treatment of what?**
   a stomach ulcers
   b anxiety
   c irregular heart rhythms
   d high blood pressure
   e angina

5 **In what forms is GTN available?**
   a buccal spray
   b sublingual tablets
   c slow release tablets
   d oral suspension
   e skin patches

6 **If you suspect a person is suffering from drug poisoning what actions could you take?**
   a keep any empty containers
   b keep any vomited material
   c put an unconscious person into the recovery position
   d walk the person around to wear off the effects of the drug
   e encourage the person to vomit

answers

1 **a**, **b**, **d** and **e**
2 **a**, **b** and **c**
3 **b**, **c** and **e**
4 **b**, **c**, **d** and **e**
5 **a**, **b**, **c** and **e**
6 **a**, **b** and **c**

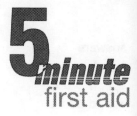
first aid

8

visual and hearing problems in later life

When giving first aid to an older person, it is important to remember that the person may not be able to hear, see or move as well as a younger person. Visual or hearing impairments are important considerations when delivering first aid to any one, but there is a specific need to be sensitive and considerate when dealing with an older person.

visual impairment

Visual impairment is common amongst older people and tends to increase with advancing age. Consequences of this can be both physical and psychological; poor sight and hearing can impact on a person's ability to communicate and there can be a sense of isolation and being ignored especially in a group setting. On a practical level, there can be an increased risk of injuries such as burns, cuts and broken bones.

If the loss of sight is sudden or severe, it can be a great shock to the person or to his immediate family. It will affect the person's mobility and personal relationships. Yet if the change in eyesight is slow, others may underestimate the extent of its impact.

When administering first aid to a person with visual impairment, explain carefully what is wrong and describe in some detail – using simple language – what you are going to do. If possible, address the person by name because this aids communication and helps the visually-impaired person to keep track of who is speaking, explain the treatment step by step and provide lots of reassurance. However, be realistic; if something you are going to do may cause discomfort, let the person know. Remember that people have different pain thresholds – what may feel like a cat scratch to one person may feel like intense pain to another.

Do not be tempted to raise your voice or shout at a person's face in the hope that they will be able to hear you better. Remain calm and remember that your tone of voice can be very helpful in reassuring a person with visual impairment.

key skills

If administering first aid to a visually impaired person, explain to the person in simple terms what you are going to do. Speak slowly and methodically and do not shout. Reassure constantly.

---

one-minute *wonder*

Q If I think a person should not be doing something because of impaired vision should I say so?

A No, do not be tempted to interfere with advice outside the scope of first aid. For example, if a visually-impaired older person has been involved in a car crash do not say, 'I don't think you should be driving'.

⑤ ● ⑤

hearing impairment

Deafness is a common problem in later life and around a quarter of individuals aged 65 and over report a problem with their hearing. It is estimated that 8.7 million adults in the UK have some degree of deafness. Of this figure, 75 per cent are aged 65 or over. Most people have a gradual and progressive loss of hearing that impairs understanding of speech and affects both ears.

You should be aware that when giving first aid to an older person there might be some degree of deafness. The presence of a hearing aid does indicate deafness, but if an older person doesn't have a hearing aid this does not necessarily mean he has good hearing. You should also remember that someone who has been profoundly deaf for a long time might have problems with speech, Give that person time to respond to your questions; it may be necessary to communicate in writing.

When giving first aid to an older person with impaired hearing, ensure that you have the person's attention when speaking, and use pointing, eye contact and touch in addition to speech. Try to have your face on the same level as the person you are talking to. Do not shout, turn away or cover your face when you are talking. Maintain normal speech volume and rhythms but speak more slowly than you normally do. Accompany words with visual actions such as hand and facial gestures, and check that the person has understood what you are saying and doing as you go along. If the person has trouble understanding a word or phrase, write it down and use clear and precise lip movements when talking to lip readers. Remember that everything can be very frustrating for a deaf person and at times their behaviour may reflect that frustration.

🌑 key skills

If administering first aid to someone with hearing difficulties, use eye contact and touch in addition to speech. Remember to speak more slowly and where possible, accompany words with visual actions.

If you are in regular contact with people with hearing problems and you are likely to have to give first aid, it might be advisable to learn how to use sign language.

British Sign Language (BSL) is regarded as a language in its own right. It is a visual language in the way it is used and understood, and it has a broad vocabulary and grammatical rules. The signs are complex and even a slight change in hand position or facial expression can change the meaning completely. It is generally used by those who are profoundly deaf and, in recent years, has formed the basis for 'deaf culture' to develop. The key components that assist communication include:

- precise hand movements
- eye contact
- clear lip movements
- correct facial expression and shoulder movements
- signing at a steady pace.

In first-aid situations, you must ensure that the person with a hearing impairment has understood you when you are:

- assessing the of level of consciousness using AVPU
- asking questions about what has happened
- giving your instructions
- explaining the treatment you are giving
- explaining what is going to happen afterwards.

difficulties with mobility

Older people frequently have difficulty moving around. This may be due to general weakness, which is a common complaint and may indicate an underlying medical disorder including arthritis (especially of the knees and hips), shortness of breath, chest pains or a previous stroke. One of the most difficult things for an older person to do is to cut toenails and, consequently, painful feet are often tolerated.

how to cut toe nails

Do not attempt to cut the toenails for a person who has diabetes or problems with circulation. Soak the feet in warm water to make cutting easier and always cut the nails straight across. Press down on the soft tissue on either side of the nail gently with a cotton-tipped stick after finishing the nail cutting. Do not try to pare a corn. If in doubt, seek the advice of the district nurse or a chiropodist.

how to help a person with reduced mobility in an emergency situation

When administering first aid in an emergency situation, you should leave the person in the position in which you found him until a medical assessment has been made. You should move the person only if there is imminent danger of drowning, fire, smoke, gunfire or falling masonry.

If you need to move a person in an emergency, it is important you do so with care using the principles described below. If you use these techniques you will find it easier for you, and safer for the person you are moving.

Position yourself as close to the other person as you can and keep yourself in a position in which you can maintain good posture. Move smoothly without jerking. In order to do this, it is best to stand with your feet shoulder width apart and with one foot slightly in front of the other. You should be aware that the older person may have mobility problems and also difficulty hearing what you are asking him to do.

If the person is able to walk, you can assist him using the following method. Stand at the side of the person, cross one hand over in front of your body and take hold of the person's hand nearest to you using the palm-to-palm thumb grip. Hold the person's hand out slightly in front of you, pass your other arm around the waist and grasp the belt, waistband or clothing at the waist. Move forward using small steps and give the person lots of reassurance as you move. Make sure that he knows what actions you are both going to take.

If at any time the person begins to fall, you risk injuring yourself if you try to catch him. The best thing to do is try to control the fall and allow the person to slide down your body.

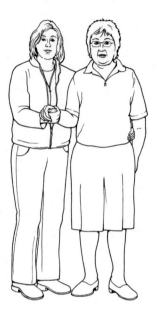

Fig 20 Walking with someone who has reduced mobility

how to control a falling person

If a person is falling, move as quickly as you can into a position behind him and put your arms out around the person but do not support him. Your arms are to stop the person falling sideways. Guide the person to fall backwards against your body and slide down your body into a sitting position. Kneel down and adjust the person's position into one that is comfortable.

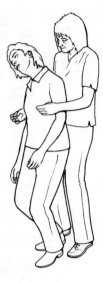
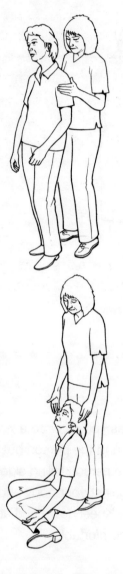
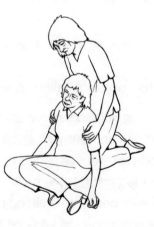

Fig 21 How to control a falling person

You can take the above actions to help an older person to move when you are by yourself and the situation is an emergency. However, you must not try to lift someone without help. This includes lifting an older person out of the bath or lifting an older person into a chair. If you try to do these by yourself, you will risk hurting your own back. You should take advice from a professional person such as a physiotherapist or occupational therapist about how to cope with an older person who is having problems with mobility. Remedial actions can be taken such as:

• the alteration of a chair's height
• taking advice on exercise
• the provision of a mobility aid such as a wheelchair, walking frame, higher toilet seat with grab rails, and grab rails at steps or to help getting in and out of the bath.

one-minute wonder

Q How should an older person who has fallen get up if there is nobody to help?

A Take their time. Roll over onto his front and raise himself onto his knees, grasp any nearby stable objects such as furniture and use these to support himself when trying to stand.

summary ▬▬▬▬▬▬▬▬▬▬▬▬▬▬▬▬▬▬▬▬

Loss or partial loss of hearing and eyesight are not uncommon in older people and as a result the person may feel more vulnerable in a first-aid situation. Speak slowly and clearly, and remember the importance of touch. Keep calm and offer the injured person reassurance throughout.

self-testers ▬▬▬▬▬▬▬▬▬▬▬▬▬▬

1 What is the best practice when giving first aid to a person with impaired hearing?
  a shout loudly in case the person can't hear you
  b avoid eye contact in case the person is embarrassed
  c use hand gestures to go with your words
  d use precise lip movements
  e speak more slowly than you usually do

2 What are the general principles for helping a person to move?
  a positioning yourself as close to the person as possible
  b bending over from the waist and lifting
  c adopting a good posture with your knees bent
  d standing with your feet together
  e moving as smoothly as possible

answers
1 **c**, **d** and **e**
2 **a**, **c** and **e**

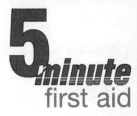

9

burns and hypothermia

In an older person with poor vision and mobility, burns are common. The skin becomes drier, thinner and looser with increasing age and so it is easier to damage and takes longer to heal. Any burn larger than a 50 pence piece should be taken seriously. There is also an increased risk of infection in an older person and you should remember that burns can be extremely painful and their seriousness is often underestimated.

A burn or scald damages the skin and if severe can lead to clinical shock (see Chapter 4, page 61). When dealing with a burn you need to act quickly to try to lessen the effect of the heat on the skin and stop the heat from spreading. You also need to keep the burnt area as clean as possible to reduce the chance of infection.

⑤ ● ⑤

burns

Burns can be superficial, partial thickness or full thickness. A superficial burn involves only the outer layer of the skin, and a partial thickness burn involves the outer layer of the skin but includes blistering. A full thickness burn involves all the layers of the skin and there may be damage to blood vessels and nerves. In full thickness burns, damage to the nerves leads to loss of pain sensation, and the skin looks waxy and charred.

how would you recognize a burn

The following factors will help you to recognize a burn:

- history of the incident
- pain if the surface of the skin is involved
- no pain if the burn is deep and has involved all the layers of the skin
- rapid swelling of the burnt area
- redness around the burnt area
- blistering.

---

one-minute wonder

Q Should I apply butter to a burn?

A No, because it is likely to introduce organisms that can lead to infection later.

If a person has suffered a burn, cool the burn with copious amounts of cool water until the burning feeling eases. Remove anything that might cause a restriction when the area swells, such as rings or bracelets. Remove any local burnt clothing unless it is sticking to the burn. When the burnt area is cool, cover it to prevent infection. For this, you can use a clean cloth, cling film, a plastic bag or sterile dressing. Arrange for the person to have further medical assessment of the burn, however insignificant it looks. If the person has been burnt in a fire, watch out for breathing difficulties from smoke inhalation.

how to apply a clean dressing to a burn

If you have access to a pair of clean disposable gloves, wear them and make sure the dressing you have ready is large enough to cover the entire burn. Secure the dressing in place with a bandage rolled gently over it, and secure the bandage with a bandage clip or safety pin.

When dealing with burns you should not apply lotions or creams as they might introduce infection. Avoid applying sticky tape or plasters to the skin around a burn as it might tear the skin. Do not burst any blisters as this might introduce infection. You should not remove any clothing sticking to the burn because this will tear the skin. Do not touch the burnt area as you might introduce infection from your hands, and do not overcool the burn as you might induce hypothermia and worsen clinical shock.

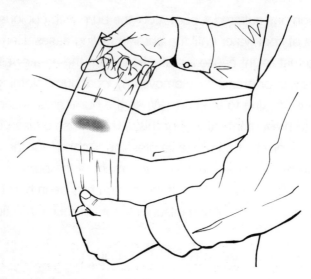

Fig 22 How to dress a burn using cling film

🕐 *key skills*

To cool a burn, place it under cool running water until the burning eases; this can take at least ten minutes. Cover with a clean dressing or with cling film.

🔵 ● 🔵

hypothermia

Hypothermia is a condition that develops when the core body temperature falls below 35ºC (95ºF). It is a dangerous condition because if it is not reversed, hypothermia can lead to slow, weakening heart activity and eventual death.

Hypothermia may result from overcooling a significant burn, but in an older person is more likely to develop slowly over a number of days. It is related to poor heating, poor nutrition, poor mobility and chronic illness.

If you suspect hypothermia, rewarm the person gradually. It is always tempting to take quick action, but that can be dangerous because of redirection of the blood circulation to the vital organs. Assist the person to move into a warmer area or increase the room temperature slowly; cover the person with warm clothing or a blanket. Do not give him a hot drink, instead give a warm drink like soup and quick-release high-energy food such as chocolate. Always get some medical assistance because hypothermia can disguise or accompany another illness such as a stroke, a heart attack or underactivity of the thyroid gland.

When dealing with hypothermia, do not allow an older person to try to rewarm by having a hot bath because this will lead to dangerous redirection of the blood circulation. Warm water should be used for the purpose of bathing the person. Do not place any heat sources such as fires or hot-water bottles next to the person as these will lead to dangerous redirection of the blood circulation and may cause skin burns. Avoid giving the person hot brandy or other alcohol as alcohol causes the blood vessels to dilate and more heat will be lost through the skin. Do not handle the person roughly because in severe cases of hypothermia rushed treatment or movement can cause the heart to stop.

key skills

If you suspect a person to have hyporthermia, rewarm him slowly using warm clothing or blankets and warm the temperature in the room. Give him a warm drink or chocolate.

---

one-minute wonder

Q Is it OK to give alcohol to a person suffering from hypothemia?

A No, alcohol can make the condition worse and there is no medical evidence of its benefits.

summary

As people get older the mobility, sensitivity and dexterity of their hands decreases. This results in burns and scalds. However, because of older people's decreased mobility, this may delay the cooling of the affected area. It is therefore important to remember that if you cannot take the person to the cold, running water, take the water to the person.

self-testers

1 When dealing with a burn your should treat it by:
    a applying butter
    b cooling it with cool, running water
    c putting on a plaster
    d removing adherent clothing
    e covering with cling film

2 **The management of a burn on the hand includes:**
  a cooling it with cool, running water
  b putting it in a plastic bag after cooling
  c popping the blisters
  d applying a skin moisturizer
  e removing all rings

3 **'Do nots' when treating burns include:**
  a application of creams and lotions
  b touching the burn to make an assessment
  c causing hypothermia by overcooling
  d covering it with a clean, tea towel
  e leaving blisters intact

4 **What is the best practice for rewarming an old person who is suffering from hypothermia?**
  a rewarm as quickly as possible using a hot-water bottle
  b if possible help the person to have a warm bath
  c slowly raise the room temperature
  d give very hot drinks
  e rush the person into a hot room

answers
1 **b** and **e**
2 **a**, **b** and **e**
3 **a**, **b** and **c**
4 **b** and **c**

Roger's story

Roger and his wife Jean had often talked about going on a first-aid course, but they both had busy lives, children to bring up, and they both worked full time. Although they were now in their sixties, their lives remained hectic and fulfilling. The dog still needed to be walked and Roger's mother lived close by and he kept an eye on her. He tended to pop in every other day for a quick chat and cup of tea. She lived alone and remained fiercely independent to the point of being stubborn. She was a proud woman who never forgot family birthdays and, like many of her age, she spent the long winter evenings watching TV and reading, interspersed with the occasional doze in her favourite chair.

Roger's mother had good general health, and despite a few of the illnesses and ailments one associates with old age, she showed the energy and enthusiasm of a much younger woman. One morning in early November 1994 was like any other. Roger let himself in to his mother's house, announcing his arrival as usual so she wouldn't become alarmed. She didn't always reply because his arrival often interrupted her 'power nap', as her family humorously referred to it. Arriving in her sitting room, Roger became suspicious that all was not well. His mother was not in her chair and he knew she rarely had a 'lie in'. He immediately went to the kitchen where he found her slumped against the door in a half sitting position. She was moaning and appeared to be in pain. Roger, while relieved that his mother was alive, could not bear to see his dear old mum in such an undignified way. A woman who led a proud existence was reduced to lying on the cold floor, semi-clothed and clearly in some discomfort. All she wanted her son to do was to put her back in her chair.

As Roger lifted his mother off the floor, there was no evidence that this increased her discomfort. He gently lowered her onto the chair and covered her with a blanket. He briefly spoke with her and, although she appeared fine, she began complaining of a slight twinge in her hip. He thought he should play it safe and call an ambulance.

Once in hospital. Roger's mother was diagnosed with a fractured neck of femur. Her condition became life threatening after surgery but she went on to make a full recovery. It was only after the accident that the family became aware of how it had happened. She was simply leaning against the connecting door between the hallway and the kitchen, not realizing the door was open, and she lost her balance and fell onto the floor.

In the weeks after the event, Roger went through a whole range of emotions: guilt that the accident had happened and that he didn't know what to do; concern that his actions may have made the fracture worse; anxiety while waiting to see if his mum was going to recover.

the authors' observations

Roger's arrival on the scene probably saved his mother's life. He didn't do anything typically heroic. On lifting her from the floor, he did recognize that his mum was not her 'usual self ' and he tried to make her comfortable and warm. Most importantly, he called for the ambulance. Without wishing to sound 'wise after the event', it is not advisable to move a person with a suspected leg or hip injury. The femur is a large bone surrounded by big blood vessels and any unnecessary movement should be avoided. If Roger had had a greater level of first-aid knowledge, he would have known that the pain in the hip area, the unnatural position of the leg, the fact that the foot was rotated further than you would expect, and the possibility that the injured leg may be shorter than the good one indicated that this was a serious injury. He might even have suspected a fracture of the hip.

Mark's story

Mark and his partner had popped in to see his Mum on their way home. On arriving at the T-junction at the end of her road, Mark noticed that a car had just crashed into a stone wall that ran alongside the road. Mark pulled up behind the accident, put his hazard lights on and, before he could get out of car, he saw an older man trying to get out of the driver's door of the crashed car. Mark spoke to the driver of the car, who said he was all right. On looking into the front of the car, Mark could see that the impact had inflated the driver's air bag. Then he noticed that there were three older passengers in the car. One of the ladies in the back was complaining of a painful leg; another appeared to have damaged her arm; and the gentleman in the passenger's seat in the front was complaining of pain in his lower abdomen. In the meantime, Mark's partner had called for the emergency services.

As there was no risk to the passengers from other road users, Mark advised all the occupants to remain in the car and to avoid moving if possible. All the occupants were responding to Mark so he knew that none of them was unconscious. The lady with the injured arm seemed as comfortable as possible, supporting it herself.

the authors' observations

Mark and his partner did a very good job. They ensured that the scene was as safe as possible by positioning their car and putting the hazard warning lights on. On this occasion none of those involved would have benefited from being moved from the vehicle. This is a very good example of 'psychological first aid'. Once they had done all the practical first aid, Mark and his partner continued to talk and reassure the occupants until the emergency services arrived.

first-aid kit contents

There are no hard and fast rules about what should be in your personal first-aid kit. What you are most likely to need will depend on where you are and what you are doing. You may wish to keep a kit at home, another in your car, and perhaps a small version to take with you on holidays, etc. It is vital that you have the necessary supplies ready to hand for when you need them.

There are some core items that we recommend you have in any kit:

- **plasters in assorted sizes** – these are applied to small cuts and grazes. Covering the wound with a clean, dry dressing will help prevent the area from becoming infected as well as help to stop any bleeding.
- **sterile wound dressings in assorted sizes** – these are used for wounds such as cuts or burns. Place the dressing pad over the injured area, making sure that the pad is larger than the wound. Then wrap the roller bandage around the limb to secure it.
- **triangular bandages** – commonly used for slings, these are strong supportive bandages. If they are sterile then they can also be used as dressings for wounds and burns.
- **safety pins** – useful for securing crêpe bandages and triangular bandages.

- **adhesive tape** – useful to hold and secure bandages comfortably in place. Some people are allergic to the adhesive, but hypoallergenic tape is available.
- **non-alcoholic cleansing wipes** – useful for cleaning cuts and grazes. They can also be used to clean your hands if water and soap are not available.
- **roller bandages** – used to give support to injured joints, to secure dressings in place, to maintain pressure on them, and to limit swelling.
- **disposable gloves** – these single-use gloves are an important safety measure to avoid infecting wounds as well as to protect you.
- **scissors** – using a round-ended pair of scissors will not cause injury and will make short work of cutting dressings or bandages to size. It is useful to have a strong pair that will cut through clothing.
- **sterile gauze swabs** – these can be used to clean around a wound or in conjunction with other bandages and tape to help keep wounds clean and dry.
- **burn gel** – use directly on a burn to cool and relieve the pain of minor burns and to help prevent infection. Very useful if water is not available.
- **ice pack** – cooling an injury and the surrounding area can reduce swelling and pain. Always wrap an ice pack in a dry cloth and do not use it for more than ten minutes at one application.
- **tweezers** – useful for picking out splinters.

- **thermometer** – used to assess the body temperature. There are several different types including the traditional glass mercury thermometer and digital thermometer, as well as the forehead thermometer and the ear sensor. Normal body temperature is 37°C.
- **face shield or pocket mask** (a hygiene shield for giving rescue breaths) – these are plastic barriers with a reinforced hole to fit over the injured person's mouth. Use the shield to protect you and the person from infections when giving rescue breaths.
- **note pad and pen** – use the pad to record any information about the person that may be of use to the emergency services when they arrive. For example, the name and address of the person, how the accident occurred, and any observations. It is also useful to record vital signs so that you can monitor how well the person is doing over a period of time.
- **basic first-aid information** – a basic guide to first-aid tips and emergency information (you can use the pull-out essential notes in this book).

This is not an exhaustive list and there are many more items you may find useful to add to your kit.

Many people like to keep items such as antiseptic cream in their kits. The British Red Cross does not include anything which may no longer be sterile after the first use due to the risk of infection and allergies.

It is easy to make your own first-aid kit by collecting these items or, alternatively, you could simply buy a complete kit. For more information on British Red Cross kits, visit **www.redcross.org.uk/firstaidproducts** or call 0845 601 7105.

The Health and Safety Executive (HSE) is responsible for the regulation of almost all the risks to health and safety arising from work activity in Britain. HSE regulations concerning kit contents do apply to employers. For more information about first-aid kits and training for the workplace, visit **www.redcrossfirstaidtraining.co.uk** or call 0870 170 9110.

household first-aid equipment

Throughout this book we have made reference to the importance of having first-aid skills, knowledge and equipment. In terms of equipment, we recommend you have a well-stocked first-aid kit (see page 144), but we also recognize that there are emergency situations where you will not have access to any of the equipment. In such situations you will have to be creative and use whatever equipment is available to you. In this section we have identified some of the items most of us already have in our homes and suggest how they can be useful in a first-aid situation.

- **beer** – you may not always have access to cold running water when treating a burn or scald. In this case, use some other cold liquid like beer, soft drink or milk. The aim is to cool the burnt area as quickly as possible using whatever cold liquid is available. Beer can be used to cool the area while waiting for water or while walking the person to a supply of cold running water. Remember, the area should be cooled for at least ten minutes for the treatment to be effective.
- **chair** – a chair has numerous first-aid uses; when treating a nosebleed, sit the person down while pinching the nose and tilting the head forward. If you are treating a bleed from a serious wound to the leg, you should lay the person down and raise the leg above the level of the heart. A chair is ideal for this purpose.

- **chocolate** – chocolate can be given to a conscious person who is diabetic and having a hypoglycaemia attack known as a "hypo". This can help raise the person's blood sugar. Chocolate can also be given to a person with hypothermia as high-energy foods will help to warm them up.
- **cling film** – cling film can be used to wrap around a burn or a scald once it has cooled. It is an ideal covering as it does not stick to the burn. It also keeps the burnt area clean and because it is transparent, you can continue to monitor the burn without removing the covering.
- **credit card** – when an insect sting is visible on the skin, a credit card can be used to scrape it away. Using the edge of the credit card, drag it across the skin. This will remove the sting. Using a credit card is preferable to using a pair of tweezers as some stings contain a sac of poison and if the sting is grasped with tweezers you may inject the sac of poison into the skin. If you do not have a credit card you can use the back of a kitchen knife or any other object similar to a credit card.
- **food bag** – a clean freezer or sandwich bag makes an ideal cover for a burn or scald to the hand. The injured part should be placed in the bag once the cooling has finished. By placing it in the bag you reduce the risk of infection and it also helps reduce the level of pain.
- **frozen peas** – frozen peas or other frozen small fruit and vegetables can be used to treat a sprain or strain. Wrap the peas in a tea towel or something similar and place them onto the injury. This will help to reduce pain and swelling. Peas are

ideal as they can be moulded around the injury more easily than bigger fruit and vegetables.

- **milk** – if an adult tooth is dislodged and cannot be placed back in its socket, it should be placed in a container of milk. This will stop it drying out and increase the possibility of it being successfully replanted by a dental surgeon.

- **paper bag** – a panic attack often results in a person hyperventilating (breathing very quickly). Reassure him and get him to breath into a paper bag, this will help to regulate and slow down the breathing.

- **steam** – if a person has a severe cough run the tap in the bathroom to create a steamy atmosphere, this may help to relieve the symptoms.

- **vinegar** – if a person is stung by a tropical jellyfish, pour vinegar over the site of the sting. This will help to stop the poison spreading around the body.

- **water** – cold running water is the preferred treatment for burns and scalds. Place the burn under a cold water tap as quickly as possible and leave it there for at least ten minutes.

- **Yellow Pages and a broom** – in the event of having to provide assistance to a person with an electrical injury, where they are attached to the current, you can stand on a copy of the Yellow Pages to insulate yourself from an electrical shock. You should then move the electrical cable away using a dry piece of wood, a broom handle is ideal.

about the Red Cross

the British Red Cross and the International Red Cross and Red Crescent Movement

The British Red Cross is a leading UK charity with 40,000 volunteers working in almost every community. We provide a range of high-quality services in local communities across the UK every day. We respond to emergencies, train first aiders, help vulnerable people regain their independence, and assist refugees and asylum seekers.

The British Red Cross is part of the International Red Cross and Red Crescent Movement, the world's largest independent humanitarian organization. This movement comprises three components: the International Committee of the Red Cross (ICRC); the International Federation of Red Cross and Red Crescent Societies; and 181 National Red Cross and National Red Crescent Societies around the world.

As a member of the International Red Cross and Red Crescent Movement the British Red Cross is committed to, and bound by, its Fundamental Principles:

- Humanity
- Impartiality
- Neutrality
- Independence.
- Voluntary service
- Unity
- Universality

the International Committee of the Red Cross

Based in Geneva, Switzerland, the ICRC is a private, independent humanitarian institution, whose role is defined as part of the Geneva Conventions. Serving as a neutral intermediary during international wars and civil conflicts, it provides protection and assistance for civilians, prisoners of war and the wounded, and provides a similar function during internal disturbances.

To find out more, visit **www.icrc.org**

the International Federation of Red Cross and Red Crescent Societies

Also based in Geneva, the Federation is a separately constituted body that co-ordinates international relief provided by National Societies for victims of natural disasters, and for refugees and displaced persons outside conflict zones. It also assists Red Cross and Red Crescent Societies with their own development, helping them to plan and implement disaster preparedness and development projects on behalf of vulnerable people in local communities.

To find out more visit **www.ifrc.org**

National Red Cross and National Red Crescent Societies

In most countries around the world, there exists a National Red Cross or Red Crescent Society. Each Society has a responsibility to help vulnerable people within its own borders, and to work in conjunction with the Movement to protect and support those in crisis worldwide.

To find out more about the British Red Cross, visit www.redcross.org.uk

taking it further ▬▬▬▬▬▬▬

useful addresses

Action on Elder Abuse
Aims to prevent the abuse of older people by raising awareness,
encouraging education, promoting research and collecting and
disseminating information.
www.elderabuse.org.uk/
Astral House, 1268 London Road, London, SW16 4ER
Tel: 020 8765 7000
Fax: 020 8679 4074
Email: enquiries@elderabuse.org.uk

Age Concern
The UK's largest organization working with and for older people.
www.ace.org.uk/
Age Concern England, Astral House, 1268 London Road,
London, SW16 4ER
Tel: 020 8765 7200

Alzheimer's Society
Provides information, support, tips and news for carers and
those affected by Alzheimer's and dementia (UK-based).
www.alzheimers.org.uk/
Alzheimer's Society, Gordon House, 10 Greencoat Place,
London, SW1P 1PH
Tel: 020 7306 0606
Fax: 020 7306 0808

Arthritis Care
Provides information and advice about arthritis.
www.arthritiscare.org.uk
Arthritis Care, 18 Stehenson Way, London, NW1 2HD
Tel: 020 7380 6500
Fax: 020 7380 6505

Contact the Elderly
Contact the Elderly groups organize gatherings for frail, older
people who live alone.
www.contact-the-elderly.org
15 Henrietta Street, Covent Garden, London, WC2E 8QG
Te: 0800 716 543

Help the Aged
Working to influence key decisions and to ensure that older
people's issues are kept at the forefront of regional planning.

England
207–21 Pentonville Road, London, N1 9UZ
Tel: 020 7278 1114
Fax: 020 7278 1116
Email: info@helptheaged.org.uk

Scotland
11 Granton Square, Edinburgh, EH5 1HX
Tel: 0131 551 6331
Fax: 0131 551 5415
Email: infoscot@helptheaged.org.uk

Wales
12 Cathedral Road, Cardiff, CF11 9LJ
Tel: 02920 346 550
Fax: 02920 390 898
Email: infocymru@helptheaged.org.uk

Mental Health in Later Life
Provides information, discussion and debate relating to mental
health. Includes the Dementia Learning Network.
www.mhilli.org
Mental Health Foundation, 7th Floor, 83 Victoria Street,
London, SW1H 0HW
Tel: 020 7802 0316
Fax: 020 7802 0301

NHS Direct
www.nhsdirect.nhs.uk
Tel: 0845 4647

NHS immunization information
www.immunisation.nhs.uk

The Parkinson's Disease Society
www.parkinsons.org.uk
PDS National Office, 215 Vauxhall Road, London, SW1V 1EJ
Tel: 020 7931 8080
Fax: 020 7233 9908/020 7963 9360
Email: enquiries@parkinsons.org.uk

Preventing Falls – Department of Trade and Industry (DTI)
Provides information and advice on preventing accidental falls within the home.
www.preventinghomefalls.gov.uk/
DTI Enquiry Unit, 1 Victoria Street, London
Tel: 020 7215 5000 or 020 7215 6740

The Princess Royal Trust for Carers
The largest provider of comprehensive carers' support services in the UK.
www.carers.org/home
London Office, 142 Minories, London, EC3N 1LB
Tel: 020 7480 7788
Fax: 020 7481 4729
For all other enquiries email: help@carers.org

Glasgow Office, Campbell House, 215 West Campbell Street, Glasgow, G2 4TT
Te: 0141 221 5066
Fax: 0141 221 4623
Email: infoscotland@carers.org

Northern Office, Suite 4, Oak House, High Street, Chorley, PR7 1DW
Tel: 01257 234 070
Fax: 01257 234 105
Email: infochorley@carers.org

Royal National Institute of the Blind
www.rnib.org.uk
105 Judd Street, London, WC1H 9NE
Tel: 020 7388 1266
Fax: 020 7388 2034

Royal National Institute of the Deaf
www.rnid.org.uk
19–23 Featherstone Street, London, EC1Y 8SL
Tel: 0808 808 0123
Textphone: 0808 808 9000
Fax: 020 7296 8199
Email: informationline@rnid.org.uk

Rukba
The Royal United Kingdom Beneficent Association is a national
charity that champions independence for older people.
www.rukba.org.uk
Rukba, 6 Avonmore Road, London, W14 8RL
Tel: 020 7605 4200
Fax: 020 7605 4201

Stroke Association
The Stroke Association provides support for people who have
had strokes, their families and carers.
www.stroke.org.uk/
The Stroke Association, 240 City Road, London, EC1V 2PR
Tel: 020 7566 0300
Fax: 020 7490 2686
National Stroke Helpline: 0845 30 33 100
Email: info@stroke.org.uk

Stroke Survivors

An informational website for victoms of stroke and their families, etc.

www.stroke-survivors.co.uk

Universal Beneficent Socity

The Universal Beneficent Socity (UBS) is a charity which helps older people in the UK who are living on very low incomes.

www.u-b-s.org.uk
6 Avonmore Road, London, W14 8RL
Tel: 020 7605 4263
Fax: 020 7605 4201
Email: ubs@rukba.org.uk

World Health Organization

Health advice on ageing.

www.who.int/topics/ageing/en

Ageing and Life Course programme
Department of NCD Prevention & Health Promotion
World Health Organization, Avenue Appia 20, 1211 Geneva 27
Fax: +41 22 791 4839
activeageing@who.int

International Red Cross contact details

Australia
National Office, 155 Pelham Street, 3053 Carlton VIC
Tel: switchboard (61) (3) 93451800
Fax: (61) (3) 93482513
E-mail: redcross@nat.redcross.org.au
www.redcross.org.au

Canada
170 Metcalfe Street, Suite 300 Ottawa, Ontario K2P 2P2
Tel: (1) (613) 7401900
Fax: (1) (613) 7401911
Telex: CANCROSS 05-33784
E-mail: cancross@redcross.ca
www.redcross.ca

Hong Kong
3 Harcourt Road, Wanchai, Hong Kong
Tel: (852) 28020021
E-mail: hcs@redcross.org.hk
www.redcross.org.hk

India
Red Cross, Building 1, Red Cross Road, 110001 New Delhi
Tel: (91) (112) 371 64 24
Fax: (91) (112) 371 74 54
E-mail: indcross@vsnl.com
www.indianredcross.org

Malaysia
JKR 32, Jalan Nipah, Off Jalan Ampang, 55000 Kuala Lumpur
Tel: (60) (3) 42578122/42578236/42578348/
42578159/42578227
Fax: (60) (3) 42533191
E-mail: mrcs@po.jaring.my
www.redcrescent.org.my

New Zealand
69 Molesworth Street, Thorndon, Wellington
Tel: (64) (4) 4723750
Fax: (64) (4) 4730315
E-mail: national@redcross.org.nz
www.redcross.org.nz

Singapore
Red Cross House, 15 Penang Lane, 238486 Singapore
Tel: (65) 6 3360269
Fax: (65) 6 3374360
E-mail: redcross@starhub.net.sg
www.redcross.org.sg

South Africa
1st Floor, Helen Bowden Building, Beach Road, Granger Bay,
8002 Cape Town
Tel: (27) (21) 4186640
Fax: (27) (21) 4186644
E-mail: sarcs@redcross.org.za
www.redcross.org.za

Taiwan and China
No: 8 Beixingiao Santiao, Dongcheng, East City District, 100007
Beijing
Tel: (86) (10) 84025890
Fax: (86) (10) 6406 0566/9928
E-mail: rcsc@chineseredcross.org.cn
www.redcross.org.cn

index